Fixing Our Broken Health Care System

By Charles Scott

Printed in the United States of America
by Mountain States Lithographing
Casper, Wyoming

International Standard Book Number 0-892944-14-6

Published by Endeavor Books-Mountain States Litho
133 S. McKinley
Casper, WY 82601
(307) 234-9325
fax: (307)-237-9521
toll free: 1-800-548-9340
E-mail: msl@mtstlitho.com
www.mtstlitho.com

TABLE OF CONTENTS

INTRODUCTION

The American health care system is entering a crisis. Its costs are growing at a rate we cannot live with very long. People are losing their health coverage as employers drop coverage due to the cost increases, or shift their burdens to their employees. Medical errors are killing thousands of us every year. Malpractice problems are plaguing many states. The combination of these factors is going to force major structural changes on the health care system.

This book is dedicated to the proposition that if we understand what is happening to our health care system and why, we can manage the necessary changes and produce much better results. By "we" I mean all of us, including not only government policy makers, providers and private (employer) payers, but also each of us personally as we make health care decisions for ourselves and our family.

This book tries to look at the whole system because all the parts fit together and an action taken to change one part will likely have consequences for other parts.

This book does not deal with the special problems of long-term care — nursing homes and related issues. That's not because long-term care isn't important; it's because long-term care has its own special issues that I'm not expert in and because the book was getting too long.

The perspective I bring to the problem is that of a citizen state legislator who has specialized in health issues for the majority of my legislative career. The legislative perspective needs to be a broad one — we are accountable for making sure the system as a whole works for all the people we represent.

If we focus too narrowly on just a segment of the system — say the Medicaid program where we appropriate the money or the special needs of an interest group like the doctors or the senior citizens — we are failing our responsibility to the rest of our constituents and asking for trouble in an election if something goes wrong elsewhere.

Being a citizen legislator adds an additional perspective to my view of the problem. I am not personally insulated from the problems of the system by government-provided insurance as the members of the U.S. Congress are. I have to go home, earn a living, and get and pay for my health care just like any other private citizen. In my case, I run a small business (a cattle ranch) that provides health coverage for its employees, so I see firsthand the problems that causes for small employers.

A couple of cautions are in order. First, this book is not a scholarly work. I use (and try not to misuse) data and statistics, and properly footnote my sources, but I do not go into the depth that one would expect in a true scholarly work. My intention is to lay out a working understanding of the problems and recommend practical actions that can be taken to deal with them.

Second, both the system and the problems are large and complex. I absolutely guarantee the reader only two things: 1) my understanding of the system and its problems is not perfect and there are important considerations and solutions I have missed, and 2) there is no one magic silver bullet that will solve all the problems. Fixing the problems will take a series of different measures, and they will at best only partly solve the problems. Also, each fix will have consequences for the rest of the system.

We legislators spend a lot of time worrying about the unintended consequences of the laws we pass. I can tell you from hard experience that the fixes for the health care system will have unintended consequences. The best we can do is try to anticipate what they might be and avoid the worst ones.

Another thing that comes with being a legislator is a willingness to make decisions in the absence of perfect information. In any legislative session we have to decide what we are going to try to do — our constituents expect us to deal with problems now and not next year. When the roll is called, we have to vote yes or no, not maybe.

I voted maybe once when I was the deciding vote on whether to pass or kill a major telephone deregulation bill in committee. I got a good laugh from the audience and an extra 60 seconds to decide to vote yes or no (I voted yes, the bill has been law for nine years, and I'm still not completely sure I did the right thing). In a number of places in this book, I will say this is what I think the situation is even though the data is not adequate to prove it. Or I will say the accurate figure is somewhere between 20 and 60 percent, but even the low estimate is large enough we ought to do something. In the real world, we have to make decisions on the best information we have, not wait until all the data is in.

So welcome to the wonderful world of health care policy. As you read this book, please consider the arguments and counter-arguments I present, but please do your own thinking and draw your own conclusions. And what you decide does make a difference. Like it or not, you participate in our health care system. We have a free market system so what you do creates market pressure that changes what happens in the health care system. And this is a democracy so what you think changes what happens to government policy. As a legislator, I can change the details and help shape the broad outlines, but in the end what our government can do depends on what all of you think and what you will support.

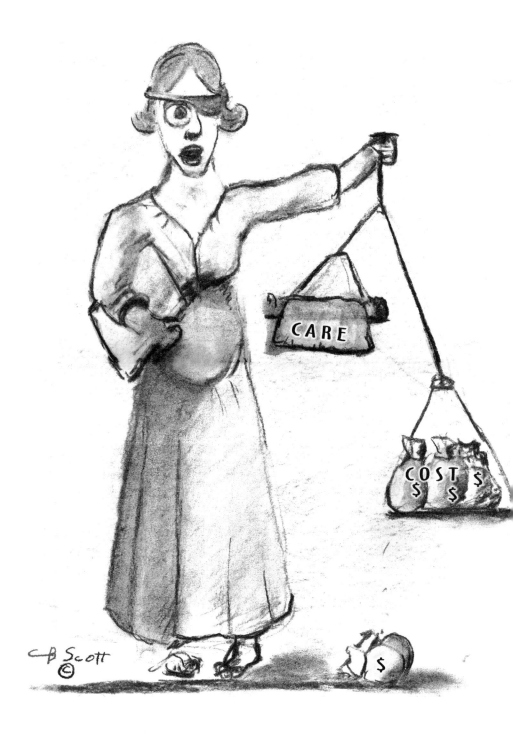

Chapter 1

WHAT'S THE PROBLEM?

We are paying too much for health care and not getting our money's worth in return.

The American health care system is in crisis. Its costs are growing at a rate we cannot sustain. The annual rate of increase for health care costs is between eight and ten percent. The U.S. Department of Health and Human Services (HHS) calculated it at 9.3 percent for 2002.[1] This is roughly three times the growth of our economy. It is a compound growth rate. A cost growing at nine percent compounded will double in slightly more than eight years.[2] This is not something we can sustain long term.

The cost growth is exaggerated in employer provided coverage. Chapter 6 on cost shifting and Chapter 7 on insurance explain why. The experience in my home state of Wyoming is typical. The nine percent annual growth rate in health costs was translated into a 27 percent growth rate for small employer-provided coverage in 2001 and 30 percent in 2002. Over the five-year period ending in 2003, the increase was over 148 percent.[3]

Nationally, the Kaiser Family Foundation and the Health Research and Education Trust reported for 2004 that family premiums in all employer-sponsored plans increased 11.2 percent while those for small employers (2-24 employees) increased by 13.6 percent.[4] No business can sustain that kind of cost growth very long.

Employees are increasingly feeling the pinch of the employers' rising health insurance costs. The same Kaiser survey reported that in 2004 compared to 2001, five million fewer jobs provided health insurance and the percentage of employers offering health benefits declined from 68 percent to 63 percent, with most of the decline among small employers. Since 2001 the premiums paid by employees for employer-provided health coverage have increased 57 percent for single coverage and 49 percent for family coverage.[5] The working men and women of this country cannot stand that kind of cost growth very long.

1

State governments are having fiscal crises that make it difficult for them to afford the increases in the health programs they run. Forty-six out of the 50 states had budget shortfalls in 2003. Excessive growth in health care spending, especially in the Medicaid program, is generally regarded as one of the two main causes of the states' fiscal problems (the other and more important one is declining tax revenues, especially for income and sales taxes).

As 2004 progresses, many states are seeing improvements in their tax revenues as the economy improves. The worst of the state deficits may be over, but the best forecast is that state budgets will continue to be tight for several years.

In the United States we spent 14.9 percent of our gross national product on health care in 2002.[6] We spend 24 percent more than anyone else and 43 percent more than our neighbors in Canada. But aren't we getting better health care for it?

No. I can't count the number of times I have heard speakers refer to American health care as the best in the world. We Americans like to believe that our system is the best at everything. Unfortunately in health care, the statistics do not support this myth. In overall measures of health care success the United States typically ranks the worst among developed countries.

Table 1 shows life expectancy at birth as of 2002 as compiled by the World Health Organization and percent of Gross Domestic Product (GDP) spent on health care as compiled by the OECD for 18 developed countries. The United States has the worst life expectancy of all the countries listed for men and tied for worst with Denmark for women. WHO also computes healthy life expectancy, which is 6-8 years less than life expectancy. For that measure the United States is worse than everyone else for men and worse than everyone else except Denmark for women.[8]

As a percentage of GDP, our health system is by far the most expensive. I use percentage of GDP because it roughly takes into account the ability to pay and some of the price level differences. We are even worse in total cost per person. Reinhardt et. al translated health spending per capita into purchasing-power parity international dollars and found Switzerland, the country closest to us, spent 68 percent per capita of what we did and our neighbors in Canada spent 57 percent.[9]

Table 1

Country	Total life expectancy at birth, 2002		Health spending as percent of GDP, 2001
	male	female	
Australia	77.4	82.6	9.2
Austria	75.9	81.6	7.7
Belgium	74.8	81.2	9.0
Canada	76.6	81.1	9.7
Denmark	74.8	79.5	8.6
Finland	74.5	81.2	7.0
France	75.6	82.9	9.5
Germany	75.1	81.1	10.7
Italy	76.2	82.2	8.4
Japan	77.9	84.5	8.0
Netherlands	75.8	80.7	8.9
New Zealand	76.1	80.0	8.1
Norway	76.1	81.4	8.0
Spain	5.3	82.6	7.5
Sweden	77.7	82.3	8.7
Switzerland	77.3	82.8	11.1
United Kingdom	75.1	79.9	7.6
United States	74.3	79.5	13.9

Sources: World Health Organization (WHO), OECD[7]

Life expectancy is at best a crude measure of quality of health care. Various lifestyle factors significantly influence it independently of health care. For example, our smoking rate is significantly less than the other countries, which should improve our ranking. Our murder rate and maybe our obesity rate hurt our rankings.

Some would argue that our ethnic diversity puts us at a disadvantage; certainly some racial and ethnic groups pull down our averages. I argue that this just shows that our super expensive system is ineffective at reaching groups that are economically poor or out of the mainstream of our society and may suffer from some lingering racial or ethnic prejudices.

With all the qualifications, the statistics say that we are not, on average, getting better results from our higher spending on health care. It is still probable that if you have certain diseases and can afford the care, you will do better in America than elsewhere. What the statistics suggest is that these advantages are more than offset by disadvantages in other circumstances.

In 1999 the Commonwealth Fund convened a working group to look at five countries, Australia, Canada, England, New Zealand and the United States. Of 21 indicators this group looked at, the United States was the best in four categories, breast cancer survival, measles incidence, cervical cancer screening rate and smoking rate (tied with Canada), and the worst in two categories, kidney transplant survival rate and hepatitis B incidence.[10] In this comparison no country was clearly better or worse than the others.

The researchers' comments on the United States are instructive: "While the United States often performs relatively well for this set of indicators, it is difficult to conclude that it is getting good value for its medical care dollar from these data. The huge difference in the amount the United States spends on health care compared with other countries could very well be justified if the extra money provided extra benefits. Population surveys have shown the extra spending is probably not buying better experiences with the health care system, with the exception of shorter waits for non-urgent surgery."[11]

Our health care system has a quality control problem and a separate medical malpractice problem. The two problems are related, although, as the next chapter shows, the relationship is different from what one might expect. The malpractice system is one of the causes of the quality problems while the malpractice crisis has many causes beyond the quality problems.

Our medical malpractice system is having one of its periodic crises that seem to occur every 10-15 years. Premiums are rising rapidly and doctors and hospitals are complaining of costs and in places are having difficulty finding malpractice insurance. In Nevada the principal trauma center in Las Vegas closed briefly and the legislature had a special session to pass tort reforms. In West Virginia the most important malpractice insurers left the state, some going out of business altogether, and the legislature had five special sessions in a year's time trying to figure out a solution. In Pennsylvania a doctors' strike was averted only when the new governor promised reforms and that crisis is still simmering. One of the largest malpractice insurers, the Saint Paul Companies, left the business entirely in 2002 and two other major companies went broke. As of April 2004, the AMA lists 19 states as in crisis.

Our health care system has quality problems. In 1999 the Institute of Medicine (IOM), part of the National Academy of Sciences, published a major report, "To Err is Human," which identified medical error as being responsible for between 44,000 and 98,000 deaths a year. If you were to put this figure into a conventional listing of causes of death, the upper end of the range would rank fifth behind heart disease, cancer, stroke and chronic lower respiratory disease and just ahead of accidents. The lower end of the range would rank ninth just behind Alzheimer's disease and ahead of kidney disease.

Some experts tell me that even the high end IOM estimate may be too low. The studies on which the IOM estimates are based are of hospitalized cases and serious errors that occur outside the hospital setting, like errors involving drug interactions.

My home state of Wyoming is like the rest of the country with respect to medical errors. In 2002 I attended a conference of Wyoming educators and municipal officials responsible for employee health insurance programs. The presenter asked the audience how many people had had a serious medical error in their family and about a third of the hands went up.

The use of a range of estimates by the Institute of Medicine indicates that there is a problem with the statistics on medical error — the experts have trouble agreeing on what medical error is and what its effect is. A family I know had an experience that illustrates this. The wife died from uterine cancer after her doctor missed the diagnosis and treated her with antibiotics for a prolonged period. Since uterine cancer is usually curable if treated early, it is probable that her doctor transformed a curable disease into a fatal one, but this is not certain. It is possible, but not likely, that even if everything had been done correctly, the disease would have killed her. Did she die from medical error or didn't she?

The problems with the statistics should not distract us from the point that we have a serious problem with medical error. Even the low-end estimates are much too high. Any comprehensive fix to the health care system needs to address this problem.

In addition to medical error, we also have a rate of iatrogenic (doctor caused) death and disease that does not arise from error. Many medical procedures, treatments and tests carry risks even when properly done. Even the normal X-rays carry a small risk — ionizing radiation has a long-term cancer risk that is well documented. Where the benefits outweigh the risks, reducing the risks is a problem for science, not health policy. Progress is steadily being made although new technology always is adding new possible risks. However, when the test or treatment is medically unnecessary and caused by flaws in our health care system, we have a problem that policy reform needs to address.

I have heard a number of health policy experts including former Colorado Gov. Dick Lamm talk about our need to ration health care to keep it affordable. I disagree. It is my thesis that if we can 1) solve the problems of medical error and unnecessary medical care, 2) stop some of the practices by professionals and providers that increase our costs without giving us value in return, and 3) use free competitive markets where they are appropriate, we can control if not completely solve our financial problems with health care. The gap between us and the rest of the developed world leaves us a lot of room to fix our problems before we have to resort to rationing that does anyone any harm.

There are those who favor a governmental single-payer system as the solution. As Chapter 12 discusses in detail, single payer is a bad solution. Due to our size, culture and politics, single payer would not work as well here as it does in Europe or Canada and it has plenty of problems there.

Others advocate other universal coverage schemes as the solution. As Chapter 13 explains, there is a universal coverage scheme financed by a four-way state, federal, employer and employee partnership that could work. It would fix the problem of our growing number of uninsured. It will not solve our cost and quality problems. In fact, I oppose trying it unless the costs can be at least partly controlled first.

There also are those who advocate free markets and personal responsibility as the solution. These are helpful but not "the solution" either. As Chapters 8, 9 and 13 discuss, a free market solution is useful in places, but the health care market is different from other markets. There are parts of the health care system where free markets will increase costs and decrease quality.

Also, while personal responsibility is useful, so many acute health problems cost so much that most people have to resort to health insurance and other third-party payers to pay their bills. For most working Americans, health care presents the classic situation where people ought to buy insurance. There is a risk but not a certainty of catastrophic costs.

If there was a single, simple solution to the problems of our health care system, it could be described in an article rather than a book.

Chapter 1, Footnotes

(1) The New York Times, "Health Spending Rises to 15 percent of Economy, a Record Level," January 9, 2004.

(2) 8 years = 1.9926 times. Source, tables in Wyoming Statutes Annotated, 1977 Republished Edition.

(3) Wyoming Insurance Department, conversations with author (January 2004) and testimony before Joint Interim Labor Health and Social Sciences Committee, August 2002. The rate increases cited were 10 percent for 1999, 18 percent for 2000, 27 percent for 2001, 30 percent for 2002, and 17 percent for 2003. These rate increases were derived to set the rates in the department's reinsurance pool and are approximate.

(4) Associated Press report, published Casper Star-Tribune, September 10, 2004, page 1.

(5) Associated Press, loc. cit.

(6) The New York Times, Ibid.

(7) Life expectancy data are from The World Health Report, 2002, complied by the World Health Organization (WHO), statistical annex, Annex Table 1, Basic Indicators for all Member States, pages 179-185. Data are for 2002. GDP data are OECD data for 2001 taken from Uwe E. Reinhardt, Peter S. Hussey and Gerard F. Anderson, "U.S. Health Care Spending in an International Context," Health Affairs, May/June 2004, page 11.

(8) The World Health Organization, The World Health Report, 2003, "Annex Table 4 Healthy life expectancy (HALE) in all Member States, estimates for 2002," pages 166-168. We are the worst of the developed countries; of course we do better than the less developed countries.

(9) Reinhardt et al., Ibid, page 11.

(10) Peter S. Hussey, Gerard F. Anderson, Robin Osborn, Colin Feek, Vivienne McLaughlin, John Millar and Arnold Epstein, "How Does the Quality of Care Compare in Five Countries?", Health Affairs, May/June 2004, page 92.

(11) Hussey et al., Ibid, pages 96-97.

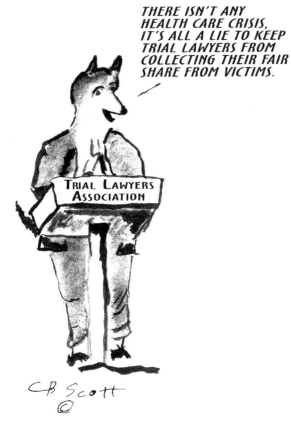
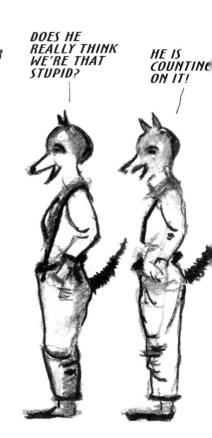

Chapter 2

MALPRACTICE

"The positions of both sides of the medical malpractice debate are well known and virtually calcified." — Health Affairs, July/August 2003, editor's prologue to malpractice articles.

None of the problems with our health care system is more contentious than medical malpractice. For the last 25 years, I have been listening to the doctors and the insurance companies saying the problem is the lawyers and the lawyers saying it's the doctors and the insurance companies. I have become convinced that each side is right about the other. We need to go beyond that sterile debate, look at what the problems really are and find new solutions.

Rising malpractice insurance rates are typically the problem that touches off the political battle. These are a source of rising health care costs although they are far from the most important source. Direct malpractice costs are generally thought to be between one and two percent of total health care costs. They have been going up faster than many other costs recently; the PricewaterhouseCoopers (PWC) analysis shows that for 2001-2002, they accounted for seven percent of the total health care cost increase.[1]

Traditionally when doctors or hospitals got a malpractice insurance increase, they grumbled, then they preserved their own income by raising their prices to the rest of us. The trouble comes because now they often can't raise their prices. Approximately half of provider revenues come from government programs, including Medicare and Medicaid, where the government sets the fees. Governments can be quite insensitive to provider requests to raise fees to offset higher malpractice insurance costs. In recent years, cutting health care provider reimbursement has been a common tactic for dealing with budget problems at both the federal and state level, and the federal and most state governments currently have budget problems.

In the proper competitive environment, managed care and even large insurers can squeeze provider reimbursement as well. When the doctors start threatening to leave an area over malpractice problems, there are usually two interacting problems — increasing malpractice insurance costs and an inability to recover those costs through fee increases.

We in Wyoming are having that problem in one of our communities right now. In 2003 the doctors in Newcastle quit delivering babies. The community is small and the doctors each were delivering between 20 and 25 babies a year. At that rate, their malpractice insurance costs had risen to over $1,000 per delivery ($38,945 with obstetrics, $12,593 family practice without obstetrics, = $1,317 per baby @ 20 babies per year).[2] Roughly half of their deliveries are paid for through the state Medicaid program, which pays $866.25 per delivery for a normal vaginal delivery; the payment increases to $1,401.87 if normal prenatal and post-partum care is provided.[3] The Medicaid program was not even paying the doctors' out-of-pocket costs.

They couldn't raise their private rates because in that community, most young couples starting a family could not afford a higher rate and too many were not covered by insurance. The economics were clear — the doctors were losing money with each delivery. They dropped the obstetric part of their practice and now a woman in Newcastle has to be driven 73 miles to Gillette, Wyoming, or 80 miles to Rapid City, South Dakota, to have her baby delivered by a medical doctor. With the distances involved, I strongly suspect many are not getting as much prenatal care as they should.

This same scenario has occurred in many communities across the country and it doesn't just affect the small towns. In many cities, family practitioners and even obstetricians with smaller volumes have had to drop obstetrics and the deliveries are done by a few doctors with a high enough volume to afford the premiums.

The malpractice crises tend to be cyclical. As explained in the subsequent chapter on insurance problems, this cycle has been made worse by the 9/11 disaster and some natural disasters that have reduced competition in insurance, generally because so much of the industry's capital was used to pay claims. Investment income has a big influence on insurance cycles and low interest income is a major factor in the current increases. In malpractice insurance, there is a long time between when the premium is paid and when the benefits are paid so the insurance company has a long time to invest the premiums.

A good return on investments can offset increases in costs. That's what happened in the mid- to late 1990s. During that period, rates were relatively stable — one of the major malpractice insurers in Wyoming even had a slight cut in rates. When interest rates fell drastically, the insurance companies had to have major increases in premiums. The related stock market decline had some impact, but most malpractice insurer investments are in interest-bearing securities, not common stocks.

The attorneys frequently blame the insurance companies for reduced investment earnings and say therefore that the insurance companies are the ones to blame for rising malpractice insurance rates. Mary Alexander, president, Association of Trial Lawyers of America, told the National Conference of State Legislatures (NCSL) 2002 Annual Health Policy Conference, "Here's the truth: the insurance industry is responsible for today's medical liability crisis. Insurance companies saw their profits go down with the stock market two years ago. They raised rates to make up for their investment losses. The insurance industry pulled the same trick in the mid-1970s and the mid-1980s."[4]

This is a misunderstanding of the way insurance works. Insurance companies get income both from premiums and from investments. The revenues from the combination of these two sources have to cover their costs for them to stay in business long term. If they can't get as much from investment income because investment returns are down, then they have to get more from premiums. If a single company has a problem because it made bad investments, the market place answer is "too bad." They've got to improve their investment performance and keep their rates down to match their competition, but that market discipline isn't available when all of the companies have the same problem with declining investment returns.

The behavior of the commercial insurance companies is instructive. They are voting with their feet and leaving the malpractice market to the physician mutuals and other carriers owned by health care providers. Saint Paul Companies, variously described as the largest (HHS) and the second largest (West Virginia Insurance Department) medical malpractice insurer left the market in December 2001. PHICO, the eighth largest, was declared insolvent in February 2002.[5] MIXX pulled out of all its states to reorganize and sell only in New Jersey, and Frontier Insurance Group left the medical malpractice market.[6] In March 2004, OHIC announced it was pulling back to its home state of Ohio and leaving seven states, including Wyoming.

An objective comment on the commercial situation of malpractice insurers can be found in the Value Line Investment Survey relative to the Saint Paul Companies. In describing the things that management had done to strengthen Saint Paul, Value Line said, "The company exited the highly unprofitable medical malpractice segment . . . ."[7]

Malpractice crises do tend to be triggered by economic factors, but economic factors alone do not account for the depth of the doctors' feelings. Being sued is never a pleasant experience — the doctors' professional competence is being challenged in a strange and public environment where the doctors have difficulty knowing how to defend themselves, particularly with the larger community. They even may well be advised by their lawyer to say nothing — something said in public defending themselves might be used against them in court.

The doctors feel, and academic studies confirm, that many of the suits are unjustified and they are being sued for bad outcomes that they were powerless to prevent. They feel that the legal system is not doing them justice. And there is always the fear, even if it rarely happens, that a runaway jury will go beyond the doctors' insurance and destroy their finances and with it their kids' college education or their own retirement.

The doctors' fear of being sued explains another problem that is very expensive for all of us — defensive medicine. Fear is not the only motivator for defensive medicine — malpractice insurers encourage it for their own financial protection, but fear is the primary motivator.

A practicing obstetrician once explained one part of defensive medicine to me. "Every woman," he said, "who needs a hysterectomy gets a bladder function study. She doesn't need it — the surgery has nothing to do with bladder function. But a percentage of the women who need hysterectomies also have bladder problems. In a few cases where these were not documented ahead of time, lawyers were able to convince juries that the surgery caused the problem. Therefore all women facing hysterectomies get bladder function studies." Unnecessary and expensive from the woman's point of view, absolutely necessary from the doctor's.

Other obstetricians have told me a bladder function study before hysterectomy is not something they do; its probably a reaction to something that happened to my source or someone he knew, but it illustrates the sort of thing that happens.

It is hard to document how much defensive medicine costs us. I have seen estimates as high as 20 percent of total health care costs. The problem is that it can be hard to separate defensive medicine from reasonable but cautious practice. Is the extra test just to be on the safe side really justified? Was the MRI really needed when the doctor very likely would have done exactly the same job setting the fracture based on the X-ray? No doctor wants to imagine himself or herself on the stand in a courtroom answering the question "Now doctor, explain why you didn't take that MRI that would have shown what my client's problem really was?"

I do not know whether the real cost of defensive medicine is 10 percent of total costs or 20 percent. I suspect it is somewhere in that range although I can't even prove that. I also suspect that defensive medicine has become so ingrained in the way medicine is practiced that if we were to remove the legal system motivations, we'd still have it for a long time. I tell medical audiences that if we were to have the most effective tort reform possible, it would still take a generation to get rid of all the defensive medicine. In addition, someone is making money providing all those tests.

Defensive medicine is more than just an economic problem. Some of it is risky for the patient. An extra blood test is just expensive. An invasive procedure always carries some risk of something going wrong. Any test using ionizing radiation carries some risk of causing future problems. The risks of ionizing radiation causing cancer are well documented. Now, the risk of a single X-ray is quite small and modern technology continues to reduce it further. But some of the new techniques use a lot of ionizing radiation.

Professor William Orrison, M.D., professor of radiology at the University of Utah Medical School, told the 2002 Health

Policy Conference of the National Conference of State Legislatures (NCSL) that a single, full CT scan carried a one in 2,000 risk of causing a fatal cancer.[8] That's a reasonable risk if the doctors really need the CT scan to diagnose a serious medical problem so they can treat it effectively. It's a totally unreasonable risk if the doctor merely needs to protect himself against legal risk. Dr. Orrison fears that in 10-20 years, we may suffer an epidemic of cancer from our excessive use of CT scans.

I have to report there is some controversy about the level of risk from the CT scan and it does vary with circumstances of each individual scan. Dr. Orrison was using the figures from the Conference of Radiation Control Program Directors published May 8, 2002. Another expert, Dr. Michael Brant-Zawadzki, used the risk figure of one death per 2,500 CT scans and then cast some doubt on the risk estimates because they are extrapolations from the epidemiological data on what happened to the Japanese atomic bomb survivors.[9]

From the public policy point of view, it doesn't make much difference unless the real risk is radically lower than either of these two estimates; it's unreasonable for the patient to run the risk if the primary purpose is to protect the doctor from personal liability. It also is important to understand that giving the patient this kind of risk runs no extra legal risk for the doctor. If the patient gets a cancer 10 or 20 years later, it would be impossible to prove in court it was a particular CT scan that caused it and not one of the natural causes or some other radiation exposure.

Even though the real extent of defensive medicine is hard to quantify, it is clearly a major cause of our excessive health care costs and a cause of the differences in both cost and quality between our system and that of the other developed countries. Any serious tort reform ought to remove the need for at least the worst of the excesses.

A number of lawyers have told me that the real problem with malpractice is malpractice. They're on to something. We have a major problem with medical error in this country. The 1999 Institute of Medicine report "To Err is Human" should be a wake-up call to all of us. It reported we have between 44,000 and 98,000 deaths per year in the United States from medical error. This would make medical error at least the ninth leading cause of death and maybe as bad as the fifth leading cause.

The next chapter will explore medical error in more detail. For now it is sufficient to understand the experts believe most of the medical error is system error. The National Institute of Medicine in their summary of "To Err is Human" puts it well:

"One of the report's main conclusions is that the majority of medical errors do not result from individual recklessness or the actions of a particular group — this is not a 'bad apple' problem. More commonly, errors are caused by faulty systems, processes, and conditions that lead people to make mistakes or fail to prevent them."[10]

This is not surprising. Our health care providers have a very human motivation to do the best they can for their patients. The licensing systems do, with rare exception, enforce a high minimum level of competence. As we have learned more about our own complex biology, the systems to treat the things that can go wrong have become correspondingly more complex. And we all know systems involving people are subject to human error. Well meaning people make mistakes for all kinds of reasons — they don't understand instructions, they don't know what someone else did to the same patient or don't understand how it affects their work — there are hundreds of reasons. The system they are working in needs to be engineered to prevent these mistakes or catch them before they do any harm. To be effective, any system run by people needs a good quality control mechanism to find and fix the sources of errors.

From the error rate we see, our health care systems do not have an effective quality control mechanism. The tort liability system has been one of our principal quality control mechanisms and the error rate shows it is an ineffective quality control mechanism.

Worse than being ineffective as a quality control mechanism, the tort liability system is an obstacle to effective quality control. To find and fix system errors, the people in the system have to identify the errors and be open and honest about the circumstances leading to them. In a situation where personal legal liability attaches to errors, it is not safe for people to be open and honest about what happened. Their lawyers will be the first to tell them "don't admit anything." Hatlie and Sheridan writing in Health Affairs put it well, "Far from encouraging transparency in health care, our adversarial legal system has normalized hiding information about risk."[11]

To give one example, the doctors here in Wyoming tell me that the rate of autopsies outside of the coroners' cases has dropped to almost zero, and this is true nationally as well.[12] Autopsies were a traditional means for the doctors to learn what went wrong in hopes they could prevent it in similar cases in the future. Some of the decline is caused by better diagnostic ability before death, particularly the new imaging techniques, and some may be due to excessive self-confidence by the doctors in their own diagnostic ability. For the most part, however, an autopsy isn't safe. It might show an error and cause a lawsuit. If an error is suspected, it could provide the evidence that could prove the error in court. It's safer to bury the mistakes than learn about them. A byproduct of that is that the mistakes get repeated.

Given the size of our problems with medical error, the obstacles that the tort liability system places in the way of effective quality control are very important. Any serious tort reform must address them.

A related problem is the way the legal system can obstruct efforts to remedy errors. Not all errors are system errors. Problems still can be caused by individual incompetence, arrogance or substance abuse. The estimates I hear are that these are 10-15 percent of all medical errors. The legal system makes it difficult for other doctors to police their own and deal with these problems. We had a case in our community that made the public press where a hospital staff committee tried to discipline a fellow doctor. He hired an attorney, sued and won a judgment in part on due process grounds. This was not covered by insurance and the doctors involved had to pay out of their own pockets. After that, a number of our local physicians told me they would never, no matter what the circumstances, vote to discipline a fellow physician.

I know of another case that was never reported publicly where a hospital committee tried to restrict the privileges of a doctor who was doing surgery beyond his training and professional competence. The doctor hired an attorney and threatened to sue. The hospital committee backed down. The doctor in question continued his practices, botched a surgery, and killed a woman. Then peer pressure ran him out of town; but as far as I know nothing formal was ever done to stop him from doing the same thing elsewhere. I believe the doctor has now died.

A problem related to its failure as a quality control mechanism is that the tort liability system is not good at identifying and compensating medical errors. The evidence from the Harvard Medical Practice study is that the tort liability system misses most of the valid claims. It showed that only about two percent of the injuries due to substandard medical care resulted in malpractice claims.[13]

The Harvard Medical Practice study itself did not analyze how the claims that were brought fared through the legal system, but the researchers involved followed these and published the results in 1996.[14] At the time of publication, 11 years after the events occurred, 10 percent of the cases remained open and unresolved. The researchers got access to the confidential insurance company files. In two cases where the initial analysis showed no negligence, the insurance company files had evidence that malpractice did occur. With adjustment for this additional information made, the results show that in 40 percent of the cases where there was a payment made, there was no malpractice. Of the cases in which there was malpractice, 36 percent resulted in no payment. Of the total claims filed, only 21 percent were valid.

These results are appalling. The system misses most of the real cases and 36 percent of the real cases that did get filed resulted in no payout. In 40 percent of the cases were there is a payout, there was no malpractice. Of all the cases filed, excluding the unresolved cases, the correct result was achieved 56 percent of the time; the system has a 44 percent error rate. No wonder the system is ineffective as a quality control mechanism and the doctors feel it is not doing justice.

The comments of the researchers on what they found are instructive although couched in the restrained language of the academic researcher. "In some cases there were substantial settlements only because the physicians in question would have made poor witnesses; in others, there was a tenacious defense even though negligence was privately acknowledged; and in still others, the cases were prolonged as part of a legal strategy. Such maneuvers are accepted as part of the art of litigation. Nonetheless, they raise questions about whether tort law is the most effective system of compensating injured patient and creating rational mechanisms of preventing injuries."[15]

The reader needs to understand that although the Harvard Medical Practice Study and its follow-up are the best available on this topic, these studies are subject to a great deal of controversy. They have been used (and misused) by the advocates on each side of the tort reform debate to bolster their case. The studies have major limitations. The Harvard study was done using the hospital medical records of a sample of non-psychiatric patients discharged from non-federal acute care hospitals in New York in 1984. It was first published in the New England Journal of Medicine in 1991.

The first thing we have to say is that it is out of date; things may have gotten either better or worse since 1984. The existence of adverse events or negligence in individual cases was based on an elaborate system ultimately relying on the judgment of at least two physician reviewers. This system has been criticized as producing results that are not fully reproducible. Finally, although the number of cases reviewed was large (31,429), the number of resulting malpractice claims was small (51), so caution should be used with the resulting percentages.

For example, take the figure that 40 percent of the malpractice claims where there was an indemnity payment were cases where there was no negligence and hence no malpractice. This is a sample and not a study of all malpractice cases in New York. It is subject to sampling error. Clearly the correct figure could be 30 percent or 50 percent. Statistically it could even be 20 percent or 60 percent. My conclusion is that whichever of these percentages is correct, from a public policy point of view, the error rate in the malpractice system is too high.

All that being said, these studies were carefully done by reputable researchers and published in a well respected peer reviewed journal. They are the best we have on the subject. They show a major problem that an effective reform must address.

A further problem with the tort liability system is that it is inefficient at compensating those who do get hurt by medical negligence. The best data we have indicates that of the money spent on medical malpractice insurance, including investment earnings, about three-quarters goes to the people who run the system and only one-quarter gets to injured victims. What happens to the money? First, the insurance companies take a cut — selling costs, administrative costs and, they hope, a profit. Then the defense attorneys and their expert witnesses get a share and these costs include amounts spent on cases that have no merit and get no payment, but still must be defended. The plaintiff's attorneys and their expert witness get a share. And finally, there is something left over for the people who are hurt.

Again a word of caution about the quality of the data. The best information I have comes from a report published in 2002 · by the U.S. Department of Health and Human Services (HHS). HHS reports, "However, only 28 percent of what they (hospitals and doctors) pay for insurance coverage actually goes to patients; 72 percent is spent on legal, administrative, and related costs."[16] When I investigated this issue in 1987, I had to combine a report from the Rand Corporation[17] with information from A.M. Best (a company which collects and publishes insurance statistics) and came up with 26 percent going to the injured victim, which I then broadened to a range of between 20 percent and 30 percent.

More recently, I analyzed information submitted through the Wyoming Insurance Commissioner to Wyoming's Health Care Commission by the Doctor's Company, one of our two major malpractice insurers. It provided information on all Wyoming cases closed by the Doctor's Company between December 31, 1997, and December 31, 2002.[18] This information gave a good picture on insurance company costs, defense costs and payouts, but it provided no information on how the payouts are divided between the costs that the injured victim must pay from the settlement (expert witness fees, court costs, etc.), the lawyer's contingency fee, and what's left for the victim. I had to use a range of between 30 percent and 60 percent for the combined contingency fees and costs. The result was that the range of what the victim got on average was between 23 percent and 40 percent.

The insurance company side of this equation is available with some careful analysis of the filings that the companies make with the State Insurance Commissioners. The division of the awards between costs, lawyers and victims, however, is protected by a veil of secrecy due to award confidentiality agreements and lawyer/client privilege. Until we lift this veil, we can only estimate how bad the system really is.

Even if we take the high side estimate for what the victim gets, we can see we have a major problem. The results of a civil justice system are measured in dollars and cents — that's what injured victims get. Any civil justice system where the people who run the system get the majority of the take, and that is clearly true here, is a scandal and a disgrace. The price of justice has gotten so high, at least in the medical liability area, that the system does justice for neither side.

A further complication is the evidence discussed earlier that 40 percent of the malpractice awards go to people who were not injured by malpractice. Assume the 40 percent figure also applies to the amount of the dollar awards and apply that to the estimate that only 25 percent goes to the plaintiffs. The result is only 15 percent of the total spent on the whole system goes to people actually hurt by malpractice.

Time is also a problem; the litigation process is slow. HHS reports, "Even successful claimants do not recover anything on average until five years after the injury, longer if the case goes to trial." This would be an even more important problem if victims depended more on the legal system to meet the expenses that errors cause them. However, HHS reports, "More than half the amount the plaintiff receives duplicates other sources of compensation the patient may have (such as health insurance)."[19]

My policy conclusions from all of this are that we need a different system to help those injured by malpractice and that as we experiment with reforms, we can't do the victims much harm because they aren't getting much help from the current system.

Much of the discussion around tort reform has centered on the jury system. Lawyers defend it as one of our key freedoms and a cornerstone of our democracy. Insurance companies and doctors denounce runaway jury awards and warn that jurors sometimes don't understand the complexities of health care and sometimes make decisions based on sympathy for a plaintiff with a bad outcome rather than the existence of negligence. The positions on both sides of this argument are largely irrelevant.

When it comes to medical malpractice, we don't use the jury system much in this country. Most cases get settled before going to a jury. For example, of the 213 cases the

Doctor's Company closed in Wyoming from 1997 to 2002, no award involved a jury verdict; all awards came from settlements. In the same period, our other major malpractice insurer, OHIC, paid out $90,000 due to jury awards, probably just one award although its data submission was not clear on that point. The threat of a jury verdict does influence settlements, but another major influence is the way each side can increase the other's costs through depositions and other legal maneuvers in the run up to a possible trial.

The report from the Doctor's Company was instructive because the company reported the defense costs for each settlement (technically called Allocated Loss Adjustment Expense). There were three cases settled for $1 million each. In two of these, costs were low: $1,700 in one case, $28,700 in another, but for one, the costs were high, $146,000. The four half-million-dollar settlements showed even more variation — $13,200, $13,900, $60,900, and $282,600. These figures show that for some cases, the outcome of a trial is clear and one side or the other gives up quickly; but in other cases, the costs can get large enough to be a major factor in settlement negotiations.

Thirty-nine of the 87 cases with settlements were settled for less than $100,000. The defense costs on these ranged from tiny ($9 for a $1,900 settlement, $10 for a $25,000) to major ($112,000 for a $71,600 settlement, $52,800 for a $12,500 settlement). The tiny amounts reported are so small there must be some general review and legal costs that never get allocated to specific cases. In how many of these 39 cases did one side or the other settle for less than they should have because of the threat of additional litigation expenses? The data shows it is a factor both sides must consider, but does not show how much it happens.

So the tort liability system has multiple problems. What can we do to reform the system?

The most common reforms are the package that goes by the initials of MICRA, which California passed in 1975. The principal reforms here are caps on non-economic damages, abolition of the collateral source rule (deduct compensation from other sources like health insurance from the malpractice verdict), periodic payment of damages (pay over time instead of a lump sum), and limits on lawyers' contingency fees.

The big-ticket items on this list are the caps and the abolition of the collateral source rule. Writing in Health Affairs, William Sage reported, "Indeed, research has shown that the favorable effect of the Medical Injury Compensation Reform Act (MICRA) on malpractice premiums in California is primarily attributable to two provisions: a $250,000 cap on non-economic damages, and the admission into evidence of collateral sources of payment for the plaintiff's economic losses."[20]

The collateral source rule is important because if it is abolished, then the victim's other sources of funds like health insurance or, in case of accidents, auto insurance are used to reduce the malpractice judgment. In a malpractice case, these other sources can be half or more of the possible judgment.

Some states like Colorado have put a cap on total damages, but in most it's limited to non-economic damages. The argument is that the economic damages are real injuries that can be objectively measured and it's only fair they should be compensated. The non-economic damages like pain and suffering also are real, but they cannot be objectively measured and are the source of much of the uncertainty over a malpractice claim and the principal source of excessive jury verdicts. A problem with this is that, at least in Wyoming, some factors one would think would be economic damages can be classified as non-economic because they can't be proved. Who can prove what the damage to the potential lifetime earnings was from an injury that permanently crippled a baby at birth? Beyond health care expenses, how do you measure the economic damages done to someone who has no wages, but is retired or stays at home to raise children or care for a disabled family member?

The doctors and insurance companies say the MICRA reforms work and are the proven prescription for the malpractice problem. They point to an impressive array of statistics that shows MICRA reforms have dramatically slowed the growth in malpractice premiums. For example, Rick Nauman from Louisiana Medical Mutual Insurance Company told an NCSL Health Policy Conference in November 2002 that data from the National Association of Insurance Commissioners (NAIC) showed that between 1976 and 2000, California malpractice premiums rose on average 167 percent while those for the rest of the U.S. rose on average 505 percent.[21]

HHS reached similar conclusions using data from different sources to compare California rates to major states without MICRA reforms.[22] The Wyoming Medical Association has bombarded us Wyoming legislators with a version of these statistics and I suspect this is true in other states where the enactment of caps is an issue.

The lawyers deny the claim that MICRA is effective. They claim the improvement in California came from the passage of insurance reforms by a 1988 initiative. I can't buy this claim for three reasons: First, there is data showing a slower rate of premium increase in California and other states with the MICRA reforms comes from reputable sources. Second, the Wyoming Health Care Commission did a survey of malpractice rates in Wyoming and its neighboring states in the fall of 2003. They included all of the states that border on Wyoming, plus North Dakota, which does not. All of these states have a cap on damages; most have other reforms as well. They used the Doctor's Company, which does business in all these states, so there should be similar rate-setting methodology. They surveyed 11 classes of medical malpractice risk. Wyoming, which has none of the MICRA reforms, had the highest rates in all but two categories, Emergency Medicine and General Surgery where Wyoming ranked third. Utah, where the reforms are recent, was highest in these two categories. Third, look at what the MICRA reforms do. They systematically reduce the payout from insurance companies for malpractice cases. I can see how people can argue that the result is unjust, but I can't see how anyone can argue that the MICRA reforms don't reduce what the malpractice insurers would otherwise have to pay out. By reducing the payouts, the reforms ought to reduce the premium growth.

Another argument frequently heard against the MICRA reforms is that the malpractice insurers won't promise to reduce their rates as a result. This claim is accurate. Almost universally, malpractice insurers have said that while reforms should slow the rate of premium growth, they will not result in rate cuts and the reforms will have no immediate effect. I heard Wyoming's two largest malpractice insurers testify this way before my committee in December 2002. What the opponents of reform don't tell you is the rest of the story, which is why reforms don't produce immediate rate cuts.

When they testified before my committee, the malpractice insurers were very clear. They are skeptics, and they base their rates on their claims experience. They don't believe the reforms will be effective until they see the results in their claims experience. A major reason for this is the courts sometimes throw the reforms out or attenuate their effect. A table published by the National Academy for State Health Policy in July 2002 is instructive. It shows that 24 states currently have caps on damages, but in seven states, caps were enacted but later held unconstitutional. Thirty states have abolished the collateral source rule, but in three others, this reform passed but was later held unconstitutional.[23] An insurance company doesn't know if a reform will be effective until it has been tested in court and that takes time.

The only time I have heard a malpractice insurance company promise to cut rates in response to the MICRA reforms was when The Doctor's Company promised a Wyoming legislative committee it would cut rates 15 percent if we enacted a $250,000 cap on non-economic damages with no exceptions that could be used to remove the cap in certain circumstances.[24] Of course, The Doctor's Company had just gotten a rate increase of nearly 30 percent. And 15 percent, while useful, is not enough to solve the economic problems caused by high malpractice rates.

I personally have two problems with the MICRA reforms. First, I am convinced that some victims of actual malpractice will be hurt by not getting all of their damages covered. Second, the reforms don't solve most of the problems with the system. The MICRA reforms will not improve the percentage of the money in the system that goes to the injured victim. By limiting what the victim gets, the caps may make this problem worse. MICRA does nothing to reduce the failure of the tort system as a quality control mechanism and little to remove the obstacles it places in the way of effective error reduction. The MICRA reforms don't reduce the legal system error rate (compensation where there was no malpractice and lack of compensation were there was malpractice and a claim was made). MICRA does nothing to improve the low percentage of those hurt by errors who even ask for compensation.

MICRA will moderate the growth in malpractice premiums. There is some evidence that it will reduce the amount of defensive medicine. There is a widely reported study, known as the Stanford Study, by David Kessler, an economist and Mark McCellan, M.D., which showed a decrease of 6.9 percent in the spending on heart attacks and 10.1 percent on coronary artery disease in states with MICRA style tort reform as opposed to states with little or no reform. To quote the Wall Street Journal, "The reduced spending had little effect on re-admission or mortality rates. The money spent on defensive medicine was wasted."[25]

There is also a suggestion now that MICRA may not always be adequate to solve the premium rate problem; its effect can be overwhelmed by other factors in the insurance and litigation systems. Every two years the Center for Studying Health Systems Change (HSC) studies, 12 nationally representative metropolitan communities to track changes in local health care markets and reports its findings in a series of useful Issue Briefs. Orange County, California, is one of the communities. HSC reports, "However, HSC findings indicate malpractice insurance pressures in Orange County are similar to those in many of the other communities studied."[26]

On balance, I view the MICRA reforms as unsatisfactory, but I have voted for them in the past and will do so again if they are my only choice. With Wyoming's low physician reimbursement and our status of the only state in our region without meaningful reforms, I am afraid that as our existing physicians retire, we will be unable to recruit adequate replacements and MICRA will help fix this problem.

Some of the doctors are starting to reach similar conclusions about the value of MICRA. In October 2003, Dr. James Herndon, president of the American Association of Orthopedic Surgeons, wrote that he believed the MICRA reforms, which he call "first generation" reforms while important "will prove to be short-term in the scheme of events because they do not address the underlying flaws in the current process. Of greater importance, these first generation reforms do little if anything to address the real problems of patient safety and medical error." Dr. Herndon goes on to advocate second- and third-generation reforms using different systems for reviewing medical cases and compensating patients.[27]

Limiting attorney contingency fees is one part of MICRA that appears to help with the problem of the low percentage going to the injured party. I suppose it does, although it doesn't reach the half of the money that goes for insurance company administrative costs or defense costs. I think, but cannot prove, its real effect is to reduce payouts and defense costs by making some of the complicated cases too expensive for the plaintiff's lawyers to risk, given the limits on their fees.

The National Academy for State Health Policy chart shows that 16 states, including Wyoming, have this reform. They are wrong about Wyoming. In this area, we have a sham reform without any real effect. The history is this: In 1987, I introduced a bill limiting attorney's contingent fees. I introduced the bill late in the session and I didn't want it to go to the Judiciary Committee because too many of its members might have a conflict of interest on the subject. I asked Senate President John Turner to use it to balance the committee workload.

Balancing the workload is a real problem that the Senate President has. In any given session, there usually will be one or two committees that for one reason or another have a light workload. President Turner sent the bill to the Mines Committee, which wasn't very busy. I introduced the bill on a Wednesday and they scheduled the hearing on it for the next Tuesday. At the hearing, I gave the pitch for the bill. I was followed by Perry Dray, representing the Wyoming State Bar Association. He said that the bill was unnecessary because the Wyoming Supreme Court had just adopted a rule that had the same formula for limitations that the bill did, and waved a copy of the rule. That was easy for the committee — we don't need to waste time passing unnecessary legislation so they killed the bill.

Later when the new rule became generally available, we looked up what it said. Sure enough, it had the same limitation formula the bill would have provided, but it also had an exception. The exception provided that the attorney and his client could contract for any fee they wanted to. Since contingency fee agreements are normally a contract between the attorney and his client, this made the rule meaningless.[28] Apparently what happened was that when the bill was assigned to the Mines Committee instead of Judiciary, the lawyers thought a fix was on and the bill was going to pass unless they did something. There was a special session of the Supreme Court. It was on Saturday.[29] The rule with the loophole was adopted, the bill got killed, and I got an education on the lengths the Wyoming Supreme Court will go to protect the income of fellow lawyers.

Repeal of joint and several liability has been another popular reform. The National Academy for State Health Policy's chart shows 27 states currently have this reform, with two that have passed it only to have the courts declare it unconstitutional. In joint and several liability, all the parties at fault are responsible for seeing that the full judgment is paid. That means the wealthy ones may have to make up the share of the poor ones. This makes a lot of sense when the parties at fault have entered into some kind of a conspiracy to do the harm. It doesn't make sense for most medical malpractice cases or for most other civil suits. We in Wyoming passed this reform after a case with which the Legislature was very familiar.

What happened was that the parties with most of the alleged fault settled. The parties that were sued, but at worst had a small amount of the fault, then had a cruel dilemma. They could either settle for the relatively large sums demanded or they could go to trial and run the risk of a very large verdict. If the verdict was large enough, they could be liable not only for their share, but also for the share of the other parties above the settlement amounts. One radiologist who did everything right except maybe being extra aggressive about seeing the attending physician got the word about the X-ray results, was reported to have had to pay $300,000 to avoid this risk. In that case, joint and several liability amounted to legal extortion and denied the minor defendants any meaningful right to a day in court or justice.

Repealing joint and several liability ends an abuse of the system, saves some money, but doesn't address the major problems with the tort liability system.

Many states have created a review panel that must review all potential malpractice cases before a suit can be filed. These can either have teeth in them (sanctions like making the results of the review admissible in court) or no teeth. The thought behind this proposal is that a review panel will get rid of potential suits that don't have merit. These are of two kinds. In some cases, the plaintiffs think they have been injured and want an objective outside party to look into it. If the review panel says, "No, the doctors did everything they should have and did it right," the potential plaintiff goes away satisfied. In other cases, the suspicion is that the case is filed without proper investigation, maybe even for the purpose of obtaining a settlement that is less than the cost of defending the case.

A panel can weed out these cases. We tried a toothless panel here in Wyoming and it seemed to be helping until our Supreme Court decided it was unconstitutional. The 2004 legislative session submitted to the voters a constitutional amendment to overturn this Supreme Court decision. They approved it at the 2004 general election. This reform, while useful, does not address many of the problems with the current system.

Another possible reform is an English rule, copied after the system used in England. It means that the loser, in addition to the judgment, pays the winning side's attorney fees. The effect of this is to make it unsafe to bring lawsuits that are not well founded. The plaintiff runs the risk of having his injuries compounded by defense attorney fees. It also encourages prompt settlement of cases that are well founded. The defense runs the risk of having the plaintiff's attorney fees added to the ultimate judgment. It makes it unsafe for both sides to indulge in the strategy of running the other side's legal expenses up as a tool to force unjustified settlements.

The English rule has potential beyond medical malpractice; it ought to have a positive effect on all civil litigation. It will be hard to enact. I can tell you from practical experience, it will be opposed not only by plaintiff's attorneys but also by defense attorneys who will support other tort reforms. The lawyers understand it will reduce the business for both kinds of attorneys.

Three cautions about the English rule. First, it is only one of the differences between the English legal system and ours. We cannot expect it alone to bring the more moderate tort liability system that England has. Second, it would be dangerous to do it without a constitutional amendment and even with an amendment, a sanction for a court ignoring it or throwing it out might be in order. It will hurt lawyers' incomes and the courts do have a tendency to protect their fellow lawyers' incomes. Third, it should apply equally to all sides.

We have a special one-sided version of the English rule in our federal civil rights laws. Under Section 1983, if a person has his civil rights violated by a state or local government, the fees of the attorney successfully bringing suit against the violation are paid by the offending government. This applies even if the sued government wins on most of the items. If the plaintiff prevails in any part, the government pays the full attorney fees. Some law firms and civil liberties organizations have turned Section 1983 into gold mines for their lawyers. Jail condition cases, employment cases, legislative redistricting cases and establishment of religion cases are favorites.

The remedy I prefer for malpractice system reform would be to replace the current system with one that focuses on patient safety. The new system would apply only to health care malpractice; it would not touch other areas of tort liability. I would create a Health Care Errors Commission whose primary task would be to find and fix the causes of health care errors — in other words to re-engineer the system so errors are prevented in the first place or are caught before they do any harm. In the process, the commission would identify people hurt by avoidable error and compensate them. Compensation would be calculated as Wyoming now does in Worker's Compensation — we would pay for all of the medical expenses caused by the error and pay for other losses on a formula.

People who think they have been hurt by an error could petition the commission for an investigation and a hearing, but commission activity would not be confined to cases people choose to bring.

As in Worker's Compensation, compensation from the commission would be an exclusive remedy, meaning people could not sue the health care providers. The commission would be funded by premiums from health care providers much as Worker's Compensation is now funded by premiums from employers.

Commission decisions could be appealed to the courts, but the judicial review would be on the record of the final commission hearing and confined to seeing if the commission had abused its discretion or misinterpreted the law. These limitations on the appeal system are normal and are designed to prevent re-creation of the tort liability system at the appeal level. I recommend that the state pay for the attorneys, when needed by an injured patient, on a fee schedule the way Wyoming does in Worker's Compensation so that none of any award has to go to pay for attorneys. I also recommend that if the patient wants to protect his or her own privacy, he or she could cause any hearing, except a court appeal, to be private with the results disseminated in aggregate and in specific only to the extent necessary to prevent future errors and with identities concealed.

The commission should be made up of professionals, both health care providers and others. It would be a mistake to limit it to just health care providers and an especially big mistake to limit it to just doctors. Medicine is increasingly a team effort and the insights of professionals like nurses and allied health providers will be essential. In redesigning systems to prevent errors, the points of view of engineers, systems analysts, accountants and teachers all will be useful. Additional public representation also may be useful.

This kind of a system should remove the fear of individual liability that is a major obstacle to patient safety in the current system. Instead of having to worry about blame and personal liability, the health care providers involved could afford to be open about what happened and participate in developing recommendations to prevent the error from happening again.

The efficiency of the system should be similar to Worker's Compensation. The most recent figures I have for Wyoming is that 83 percent of the money spent goes for benefits for injured parties and 17 percent to administrative costs. I expect the Health Care Errors Commission administrative costs to be a little higher than this due to the efforts to redesign to prevent future errors.

This system ought to reduce defensive medicine costs. The providers will lose their motivation for defensive medicine and the commission could investigate the more common practices and see if they really add anything to patient safety.

For most patients hurt by medical error, this revised system should be a better deal than the current system. For starters, they could get justice without having to pay attorney fees — if a lawyer were needed, the state would pay him.

Reducing the cost to use the system would result in compensation in many cases with real, but relatively small, damages. Now these never get compensated because bringing a lawsuit for them is too costly.

A risk is that the new system will cost more. Remember the estimate that only two percent of the injuries due to substandard care now result in malpractice claims. The unfiled 98 percent includes a lot of small cases, but it also includes a number of very expensive injuries. A new system that is cheaper and easier to use will result in more claims being made and paid. Replacing a system that takes 75 percent of the money to run the system with one that should take 20-25 percent gives a lot of margin for paying more claims, but there is a risk that the new system will be more costly than the old, at least until we reduce the level of errors.

Using a panel of professionals rather than the current settlement by intimidation system should reduce the error rate. The professional panel will make mistakes; they're human. But it shouldn't be hard to do a lot better than the current 44 percent error rate.

The new system would do a better job of meeting actual medical expenses arising from an error. In a long lasting complicated case now, a jury has to estimate how large future medical expenses will be; the commission, like our Worker's Comp system, doesn't have to do this, it pays them as they occur.

How good a job is done on the design of the specific formulas for compensating economic damages like lost wages and the economic damages will influence how well injured victims do in these areas. Like Worker's Comp, there will be tradeoffs here on generosity of benefit design vs. cost to the society at large. It is safe to say that the big jackpot awards that a few people now get will no longer be available.

This new proposed system is opposed by many trial lawyers. It would cut them out of what has been an important and profitable line of business. It also implies that the legal system, the foundation of their profession, doesn't work in this important area. The result is that professional pride will be added to their economic motivation — a powerful combination. So far, the opposition from malpractice insurance companies has been limited to one agent at a committee hearing at the 2004 session of the Wyoming Legislature, but I expect more in the future. If adopted, this new system abolishes their role and puts them out of business.

New Zealand and Sweden have successful systems very similar to this proposed medical errors commission system. However, to the best of my knowledge, this new system has never been tried anywhere in the United States, although some academics and health care experts have made somewhat similar proposals. George Huber writing in Health Affairs proposed injury compensation tables and specialty courts.[30] Former United States Senators George McGovern and Alan Simpson have written, "Distrust by doctors is so great that medicine now may need a separate system of justice that can more reliably distinguish between good care and bad care."[31] Michelle Mello of the Harvard School of Public Health has advocated limited administrative (no-fault) systems that would "compensate events that meet the Swedish definition of avoidability."[32] Dr. Mello did question the political feasibility of what I am advocating — a governmental system of administrative compensation as an exclusive remedy.

In the 2003 Wyoming legislative session, Senator Tex Boggs, D-Rock Springs, and I first proposed this new system. Our proposed constitutional amendment got out of committee but was defeated by the full Senate on a 15-to-15 tie vote in committee of the whole. I viewed this result as a reasonable showing for the first attempt at a new system. The committee I co-chair, the Joint Interim Labor, Health and Social Services Committee, presented a revised and streamlined version of this proposal to the 2004 session of the Wyoming Legislature where it passed the Senate by a vote of 21 to 9, but failed in a House committee.

In July 2004, the Wyoming Legislature had a special session on malpractice because OHIC, the malpractice insurer

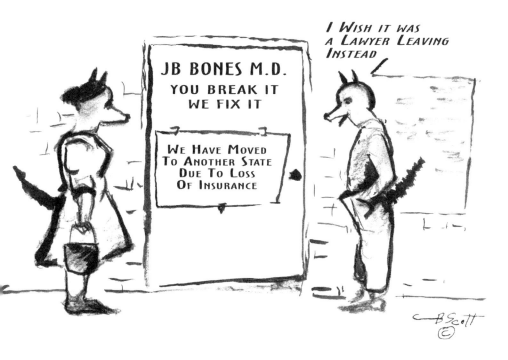

with a nearly 50 percent market share, announced it was leaving Wyoming and would stop renewing policies October 1, 2004. Judiciary Committee members were able to prevent the proposed medical errors commission reforms from getting on the agenda for the special session with the result the Legislature submitted a constitutional amendment authorizing a MICRA-style cap on non-economic damages to the voters. It did not pass the rest of the MICRA reforms. The medical errors commission reform is being studied by our Healthcare Commission.

It will be interesting to see how Wyoming's malpractice crisis plays out. At the 2004 General Election, the voters rejected the constitutional amendment authorizing the MICRA-style caps. I predict an acute crisis with the loss of major parts of our medical system. We in the Legislature will try to prevent this disastrous outcome, but we may not succeed. The Wyoming Constitution explicitly forbids the two most certain remedies. We can't reduce costs by restricting or capping damage awards. We can't directly subsidize doctors.

Chapter 2, Footnotes

(1) PriceWaterhouseCoopers, "The Factors Fueling Rising Healthcare Costs," April 2002, page 10. This document is a report prepared for the American Association of Health Plans.

(2) The rates are for the Doctors Company — obtained by the author from the Wyoming Health Care Commission.

(3) These rates were those in effect in 2003 when the doctors decided to drop obstetrics. The 2004 special session of the Wyoming Legislature held in July 2004 significantly increased Medicaid reimbursements, trying to deal with this problem. It is not yet clear whether the rate increase will be enough to return obstetrics to Newcastle. Once a service is lost, it is hard to get it back as the existing doctors will have purchased their "tail" coverage insurance and they will be reluctant to repeat that expense especially if they are nearing retirement age.

(4) Comments of Mary Alexander, President, Association of Trial Lawyers of America, at the National Conference of State Legislatures 6th Annual Health Policy Conference, Session: Medical Errors and Jury Awards; Facing Down a Crisis in Medical Malpractice, November 17, 2002, quoted from the printed comments handed out by Ms. Alexander at the session.

(5) West Virginia Insurance Department, presentation to National Conference of State Legislatures.

(6) U.S. Department of Health and Human Services (HHS), Office of the Assistant Secretary for Planning and Evaluation, "Confronting the New Health Care Crisis: Improving Health Care Quality and Lowering Costs by Fixing Our Medical Liability System," July 24, 2002, page 14.

(7) "The Value Line Investment Survey," September 26, 2003, page 607.

(8) Dr. William Orrison, MD, Professor of Radiology, University of Utah, statement contained in a presentation and the handed out copies of the slides he used, presentation given to the Annual Health Policy Conference, National Conference of State Legislatures, November 2002.

(9) Michael Brant-Zawadzki MD and Jeffrey M. Silverman, MD, "CT Screening: Why I Do It," American Journal of Radiology, July 2002; 179: 319-326, quoted by Orrison in presentation cited above.

(10) Page 2 of a brochure entitled "To Err is Human: Building a Safer Health System, dated November 1999 and distributed by the Institute of Medicine to summarize their publication of the same title.

(11) Martin J. Hatlie and Susan E. Sheridan, "The Medical Liability Crisis of 2003: Must We Squander the Chance to Put Patients First?" Health Affairs, July/August 2003, Vol. 22 #4, page 38.

(12) Atul Gawande, Complications, A Surgeon's Notes on an Imperfect Science, Picador, New York, 2002, page 191. For an excellent discussion of the other reasons for the decline in autopsies and the continuing need for them read Gawande's full chapter on this subject, pages 187-201. For information on the decline in autopsies nationally see E. Burton, "Medical Error and outcome measures: Where have all the autopsies gone?" Medscape General Medicine, May 28, 2000

(13) A. Russell Localio, et al, "Relation between Malpractice Claims and Adverse Events Due to Negligence: Results of the Harvard Medical Practice Study III," New England Journal of Medicine, 1991; 325: 245-251.

(14) Troyen A. Brennan, MD, JD, et al, "Relation between Negligent Adverse Events and the Outcomes of Medical-Malpractice Litigation," New England Journal of Medicine, 1996, 335: 1963-1967

(15) Brennan, Ibid, page 1967

(16) HHS, Ibid, page 11.

(17) James S. Kakalik and Nicholas M. Pace, "Cost and Compensation Paid in Tort Litigation," Institute for Civil Justice, Rand Corporation.

(18) Michael O'Donohue, Assistant Vice President, Regulatory Compliance, The Doctors Company, letter to Ken Vines, Wyoming Insurance Commissioner, October 7, 2003

(19) HHS, Ibid, page 11.

(20) William M. Sage, "Medical Liability and Patient Safety," Health Affairs, July/August 2003, Vol. 22 No.4, page 32.

(21) Rick Nauman, Vice President, Louisiana Medical Mutual Insurance Company, presentation at the Annual Health Policy Conference, National Conference of State Legislatures, November, 2002, reported source, NAIC Profitability By Line By State.

(22) HHS, Ibid, page 13 citing Medical Liability Monitor's "Trends in 2001 Rates for Physicians' Medical Professional Liability Insurance," Vol. 25, No. 10, October 2001.

(23) Mimi Marchev, "The Medical Malpractice Insurance Crisis: Opportunity for State Action," National Academy for State Health Policy, July 2002, page 10.

(24) Testimony of Dr. Richard Anderson, CEO The Doctors Company, before the Joint Interim Judiciary and Labor, Health and Social Services Committees, Wyoming Legislature, June 22, 2004. Dr. Anderson also said the full MICRA package would result in a rate decline of 20% to 25%.

(25) The Wall Street Journal, January 16, 1997, page A 18.

(26) Robert Berenson, Sylvia Kuo, and Jessica May, "Medical Malpractice Liability Crisis Meets Markets: Stress in Unexpected Places," Issue Brief No. 68, September 2003, Center for Studying Health System Change (HSC), page 2.

(27) Dr. James H. Herndon, MD, "Alternate approaches to medical liability reform," AAOS [American Academy of Orthopedic Surgeons] Bulletin, October 2003.

(28) The rule is still there. Rule 5(c) of the <u>2003 Wyoming Court Rules on Contingent Fees</u> reads, "The provisions of this rule are not intended to abridge the freedom of the attorneys and clients to contract for different percentages."

(29) The 1991 Replacement Edition of the <u>Wyoming Court Rules Annotated</u>, prepared under the supervision of the Supreme Court of Wyoming, lists the date of amendment to Rule 5 of the "Rules Governing Contingent Fees for Members of the Wyoming State Bar," which is the relevant rule, as January 31, 1987, effective May 5, 1987. January 31, 1987, was the Saturday between the day I introduced the bill and the day of its committee hearing.

(30) George A. Huber, "Creating a Safe Environment," Health Affairs, July/August 2003, Vol. 22, No. 4, page 43.

(31) George McGovern and Alan K. Simpson, "We're Reaping What We Sue," Wall Street Journal, editorial page, April 17, 2002

(32) Michelle Mello, presentations to NCSL Annual Health Policy Conference, November 2002 and NCSL annual meeting, quote is taken from her presentation slides passed out at the session.

Chapter 3

THE MEDICAL ERRORS PROBLEM

In the previous chapter on malpractice, I briefly discussed the findings of the Institute of Medicine's (IOM) report "To Err is Human." Its findings that between 44,000 and 98,000 American deaths per year were caused by avoidable medical error were initially controversial, but have since become generally accepted. In fact, many experts believe that they are low.

To quote Dr. Kenneth Shine, president of the IOM, "The evidence since that time [November 1999, when the report was published] suggests those numbers are actually low. It is clear in the studies that led to these numbers that in many cases errors that occurred were often not recorded in the patient's chart. Second, these figures did not include the nursing home deaths or the ambulatory care deaths. Since that time, studies of nursing homes and of the ambulatory arena have demonstrated substantial, serious problems."[1]

Other studies confirm the IOM finding that we have a high rate of health care error. Before the IOM report came out, Dr. Lucian Leape writing in the Journal of the American Medical Association (JAMA) said, "Autopsy studies have shown high rates (35-40 percent) of missed diagnoses causing death. One study of errors in a medical intensive care unit revealed an average of 1.7 errors per day per patient of which 29 percent had the potential for serious or fatal injury."[2]

With this kind of evidence of a problem, fixing the medical error rate has to be a top priority of health care reform. The most important need is saving the lives of those now being killed by medical error, but there is an economic component as well. Treating those injured has got to be expensive. What is the nature of the errors? Why are they happening? To understand how to prevent them, we need to answer these two questions.

Both Shine and Leape blame the culture of medicine. To quote Leape, "But the most important reason physicians and nurses have not developed more effective methods of error prevention is that they have a great deal of difficulty in dealing with human error when it does occur. The reasons are to be found in the culture of medical practice." Also, "Physicians are expected to function without error, an expectation that physicians translate into the need to be infallible. One result is that physicians . . . come to view an error as a failure of character — you weren't careful enough, you didn't try enough."[3]

Shine is similar, "Medicine continues to foster an aura of infallibility of the physician, and in many ways remains a 'blame and shame' type of profession in which the individual physician is supposed to know everything and not acknowledge when he or she is wrong or makes errors."[4]

How does this culture translate into practice? Leape says, "The organization of medical practice, particularly in the hospital, perpetuates these mores. Errors are rarely admitted or discussed among physicians in private practice. Physicians typically feel, not without reason, that admission of error will lead to censure or increased surveillance or worse, that their colleagues will regard them as incompetent or careless. Far better, conceal a mistake, or, if that is impossible, to try to shift the blame to another, even the patient."[5]

In the previous chapter I cited the evidence that shows most of the errors are system errors. As far as I can tell since the IOM report, the medical professional literature on the subject of errors has shown nearly complete agreement that most errors are system errors. Well meaning and well trained, but human, professionals are making large numbers of errors; a problem that could be cured by redesigning the system to prevent the kinds of mistakes people are likely to make.

Atul Gawande, a practicing surgeon, puts it very well, "Yet everything we've learned in the past two decades — from cognitive psychology, from 'human factors' engineering, from studies of disasters like Three Mile Island and Bhopal — has yielded some insights: not only do all human beings err, but they err frequently and in predictable, patterned ways. And systems that do not adjust for these realities can end up exacerbating rather than eliminating error."[6] I would add to this that human errors are only part of the problem — people can do everything right in the context of their system but get bad results if the system is flawed.

The tort liability system is part of the problem. To quote NCSL's State Health Notes, "But despite the IOM's admonition that 'this is not a bad apple problem' efforts to eliminate errors run up against a legal system focused on individual liability and personal injury." And NCSL cites Michelle Mello, professor of health policy and law at the Harvard School of Public Health, as observing, "During today's perceived medical malpractice crisis, providers may be especially hesitant to report on errors."[7] In addition, the tort liability system reinforces the culture of infallibility problem that Leape and Shine cite.

The premise behind both is that infallibility is the norm and errors are wrongdoing. The legal system punishes them as torts, seeking to add financial punishment to the personal and collegial censure the culture imposes. My judgment is that both have to be dealt with to solve the errors problem.

Let's look at some of the specific examples. Problems with prescription drugs are probably the most common errors. Doctors' notoriously bad handwriting is often cited as the cause, but the problem goes well beyond that. The Health Care Purchaser, a publication of the National Health Care Purchasing Institute, says, "The most common cause of injury to patients is adverse drug events (ADEs), which are injuries due to inadequate medication, incorrect dosage or frequency, or improper drug choice."[8]

To their list I would add drug interactions. Often adverse drug interactions happen because the patient has two or more physicians prescribing and each doctor doesn't know what the others are prescribing for that patient. Dr. George McMurtry, a member of the Wyoming State House of Representatives who for many years ran the emergency room at the Campbell County Memorial Hospital, has told my committee tales of his experience with this problem. He trained his EMTs to bring in the patient's prescription medications whenever they brought a patient from home. Dr. McMurtry said that when the EMTs brought in a grocery sack of prescriptions, he knew before he examined the patient what the cause of the trouble was likely to be.

A computerized physician order entry system is a remedy for this set of problems that is becoming quite popular. As the Health Care Purchaser says, "Many ADE cases are preventable. The implementation of a computerized physician order entry (POE) system, according to one study, has decreased the rate of ADEs by more than 50 percent."[9] A good POE will deal with the bad handwriting problem, catch dosage errors, incorrect medications, and identify known drug interaction problems. A hospital-based POE will not, of course, catch the problem of two or more physicians prescribing conflicting medications to the same patient in their office setting.

Another factor that has been associated with errors is hospital staffing ratios. In a study of Pennsylvania hospitals in 1998 and 1999, Linda Aiken and her colleagues found that each additional patient per nurse was associated with a seven percent increased risk of a patient dying within 30 days of admission to the hospital.[10] The implication of this study is that as the nursing workload increases, the risk of errors both of omission and commission increases. It makes sense that as the workload increases, the nurse will be able to spend less time with each patient and will be under increasing stress, both factors that should increase the chance of mistakes being made. In 1999, California responded to this problem by passing legislation mandating patient/nurse ratios to go into effect in July 2003.

Sometimes problems can arise from efforts to prevent problems. A colleague told me of a situation in one of our large cities in the Midwest. There were two hospital systems. They were aware of the publicity over cases where surgeons had operated on and even removed the wrong leg, a problem that can happen with our bilateral anatomy. They decided to mark the patient ahead of time to prevent this problem. With that kind of a system, all concerned, including especially the patient, can and will act as quality control and make sure the right place gets marked. Unfortunately, one hospital decided to put an "x" on the leg that was to be amputated and the other put it on the one that was not to be amputated. And a number of the surgeons had privileges in both hospitals. Fortunately someone caught this accident waiting to happen.

Sometimes it takes some analysis to figure out the source of errors. Shine tells of a New York hospital that had a very poor risk adjusted mortality rate for cardiac surgery patients in spite of having well trained surgeons on staff. Analysis showed elective patients did well in that hospital but emergency cases did not. What the surgeons had done was instruct the emergency room staff to get unstable patients to the operating room as fast as possible. Other cardiac programs were stabilizing such patients in the emergency room first before operating. It turns out that stabilizing the patients first is a more successful strategy than getting them to the OR faster, something not obvious until the results of the two strategies are compared. The hospital changed its policy and the excess deaths stopped.[11]

In this example, it took comparison of the results at different hospitals and a site visit by outsiders to identify the problem. Shine reports that the hospital argued that the mortality was high because of very sick patients and that the risk adjustment was inaccurate. This is a plausible argument — a person with an unstable cardiac emergency is very sick and at risk of dying — and the people involved were in good faith misleading themselves and missing the fact they had a classic system error. Everybody involved was doing well what the system called for, but the design of the system was flawed.

Hospitals can go a long way toward reducing errors and instilling an effective culture of patient safety in their institutions. In December 2003, I attended a presentation given by Dr. John Brody, President of Johns Hopkins University, where he related what they had done in their hospital. He gave four items that he regarded as keys: 1) set an audacious goal — zero defects, 2) make everyone responsible for patient safety (and empower them to act in unsafe situations), 3) Simplify the process for example by standardizing the steps taken, and 4) improve communication among providers.[12]

Based on Dr. Brody's presentation, I would add a fifth to that list — active commitment by the top management of the institution is essential. For example, Johns Hopkins discovered they could improve the results of cardiac surgery by having a "pre-flight" check list in the OR with a nurse assigned specifically to go through it and make sure everything was ready. The rule was the operation could not proceed until that nurse said everything was ready. Enforcing that rule took a confrontation in the OR between Dr. Brody and a senior attending physician who was not about to let any mere nurse tell him he couldn't start the operation yet.

One part of the solution to the errors problem that is on most lists is greater use of information technology. It is recommendation #9 in the Institute of Medicine's report, "Crossing the Quality Chasm."[13] A key part of this is an electronic patient records system. Halvorson and Isham state bluntly, "The next major improvement in U.S. health care will result form the carefully designed and consistent use of AMRs [automated medical records]."[14]

The health care business has lagged behind other fields of endeavor in utilizing information technology. Way out in the Russian boondocks in Kizhi near the Arctic Circle north of Saint Petersburg, I used a credit card to buy a necklace for my wife. The Russian merchant was able to swipe my card and get a prompt authorization from the credit card company. The purchase was without difficulty and showed up accurately translated into dollars on my next credit card bill.

Yet if I get hauled into the emergency room of my local hospital after 5:00 p.m., there is no way they can access my medical records in my doctor's office three city blocks away. And that lack of information could make a vital difference to the treatment I get. And the only way my doctor found out I had gotten my flu shot as per his recommendation was that I told him when he saw me on a different matter that I had gone to the Senior Center and gotten it. An appropriate part of taking care of my diabetes could have been to follow up to make sure I had gotten my flu shot, but he had no efficient way of doing that. By the time he asked during an office visit it would have been too late to have done anything if I had not already done it — by then the year's flu vaccine had all been used.

My situation is not unique. It is the norm. As of January 2004, my doctor still had a massive paper filing system which is very common. There is no electronic record system that bridges the various organizations that make up our health care system, and this is true all over the United States. Kim Slocum of AstraZeneca LP reports that less than 10 percent of U.S. hospitals and only 17 percent of physician practices have adopted electronic medical records technology.[15]

These percentages have improved since they were calculated and are continuing to improve, but we still have a long way to go. The result is that patients have to get duplicate tests because the doctors can't get access to tests done earlier, an added cost for the patient, which also may delay needed treatment. And doctors have to treat patients with incomplete knowledge of what has been done to them before, a prescription for error.

A symptom of the lack of comprehensive electronic patient record systems is the relatively low spending on information technology by the health care industry. Coye and Bernstein gathered data from a number of sources to show health care spends only 2.2 percent of its operating budget on information technology while retail trade spends 3.9 percent and financial services spend 11.1 percent.[16]

A number of unified organizations have effective electronic patient record systems. The Veterans Administration (VA) has had one for some time. It significantly improves the quality and efficiency of their patient care, but it doesn't automatically capture care provided outside the VA system. A number of the better HMOs have systems that again work well within their organizations, but don't interface with other systems to capture care provided outside their own organizations.

There are a couple of reasons why the private sector has not and should not be expected to invest in the development of comprehensive patient record systems. First, the bulk of the monetary savings accrue to the patients or their health insurance company, while the costs fall on the providers. In fact, an effective system may even cost some providers money by eliminating the need for duplicate tests. Second, there are effective commercial systems on the market that can meet the providers' internal needs, but they don't interface with other systems to provide comprehensive records.

Here in Wyoming we are exploring the possibility of an electronic patient records system. My committee proposed and the 2004 Legislature funded a feasibility study on the topic. I know a number of other states are interested. In Canada, British Columbia has a working system that covers prescription drugs and both Alberta and Saskatchewan are in the process of developing more comprehensive systems. The Canadians have a single-payer governmental system paying for most of their health care, but their delivery system is enough like ours using a number of independent providers so their experience will be instructive.

As we look at the possibilities of electronic patient records, we in Wyoming think that getting the providers to actually use the system will be key. We figure they will resist a system imposed by the government from the outside. The development of the system therefore ought to be governed by the doctors, nurses and hospitals that will actually use it so that it will meet their actual clinical needs.

A further possible use of an electronic patient records system is to generate computer prompts of diagnostic issues and treatments the doctor ought to consider. The prompts would be based on standardized practice guidelines and treatment protocols. Some think the doctors ought to know all this without being prompted, but the plain fact is that the diseases people can get are so varied and the knowledge has become so extensive that no human can reasonably be expected to remember all the possibilities all the time. It's not that the doctors don't know what's in the practice guidelines; it's that they can't remember everything on the spot because they're human too. A computerized reminder system can therefore be very useful, even if sometimes the doctor will have good reason not to follow the standard recommendations in a specific case.

Using an electronic system this way would require the development of practice guidelines, which should be based on the best scientific evidence available. This was one of the factors Dr. Paul Ellwood of the Jackson Hole Group emphasized in testimony before my committee in August 2003.[17]

A computerized system also could be used to prompt the patient to do specific things his disease should require. For example, if the records show patient X is a diabetic, the computer could send reminders to the patient to get his annual eye exam from his ophthalmologist, a key to preventing blindness, a major complication of diabetes.

Another thing the government can do is fix the reimbursement system to remove the incentive for error it now contains. Many authorities have pointed this out. Shine says, "The system itself is bizarre. If the system makes a mistake and produces kidney failure, this will put the patient into a higher-paying DRG. That is clearly not aligning incentives with regard to quality."[18] This is not to say that providers will cause errors because they get paid to fix them — nobody in the health care business is that callous. But the system does remove the incentive to reduce errors and improve care.

Shine gives the example of a group of doctors who substantially reduced their income with an improved diabetes management program because with improved management, the patients needed to see their doctors less often and the doctors were reimbursed on a fee for service basis. How many quality improvement programs are not implemented because this kind of result makes them not cost effective, at least from the provider's point of view?

Now, from the point of view of a state legislator, what can be done to reduce health care errors? Organizing and partly funding the development of a comprehensive electronic patient record system is one thing the states should do. In the absence of state action, I don't see any other organization capable of doing this. In fee-for-service medicine or an HMO that contracts with provider groups rather than hiring its own staff, no provider has enough of the business to make a comprehensive system work.

In unified systems like the VA or staff model HMO's, there is enough of a concentration of business to justify such systems and they are being used. But those systems are less than complete because they don't cover out of network providers and because when a patient switches to another HMO or fee-for-service, the record can't follow electronically.

So funding a comprehensive electronic patient records system is one thing a state legislature can do to reduce medical errors. We also can legislate on specific issues like California did on nursing staffing ratios. Overtired providers are a potential source of error — we could legislate hours of service. There is precedent for that — the hours an airline pilot, railroad engineer or truck driver can work are limited by the government.

We can try to persuade. My committee under the leadership of Senators Tex Boggs and Mike Massie is trying to persuade our hospitals in Wyoming to move to one of the proven nursing programs like the Magnet Hospital program that Poudre Valley Hospital in Fort Collins, Colorado, uses so successfully. We know that often the suggestions that legislation might be necessary will produce "voluntary" efforts that solve the problem better than actual legislation would. We have not had success yet with suggestions and are now looking at incentives we could use. If that fails, we may legislatively mandate something.

In general, however, I am nervous about legislative mandates in this area. We can too easily get into the business of legislating the practice of medicine, something legislatures do not do well and should avoid if possible. I think a better approach is to modify the health care delivery system so the system puts patient safety first. There have been a number of attempts at this, but to date they have not been very successful.

Health care is full of quality assurance committees and review committees, many of them mandated by the federal government through the Medicare and Medicaid programs. They have not been overly effective; they have been around for years and have not prevented our current error problems. I see at least two reasons they have not worked adequately. First, many have been seen as bureaucratic exercises mandated by the government rather than a vital part of health care, they are therefore given only pro-forma compliance. Second, providers have been afraid to be fully open with them due to individual liability fears.

A popular remedy in legislative circles currently is mandatory reporting system requiring the reporting and, often, publication of statistics relating to errors. The IOM, in "To Err is Human," called for the creation of reporting systems. The National Academy for State Health Policy issued a report on the subject.[19] NCSL says, "For their part, states are seeking to improve reporting of preventable "adverse events," and further reports that 17 states have in place programs that require hospitals to report adverse events, and five others have voluntary programs.[20]

These reporting programs can have value. In the New York hospital case cited above, the poor performance on cardiac surgery was spotted using a reporting system that allowed the comparison of the success rates at different hospitals. Halvorson and Isham state, "We know from the Internet-based programs HealthPartners has run in Minnesota that measuring and reporting the outcomes of care also improves care system performance." They go on to talk of

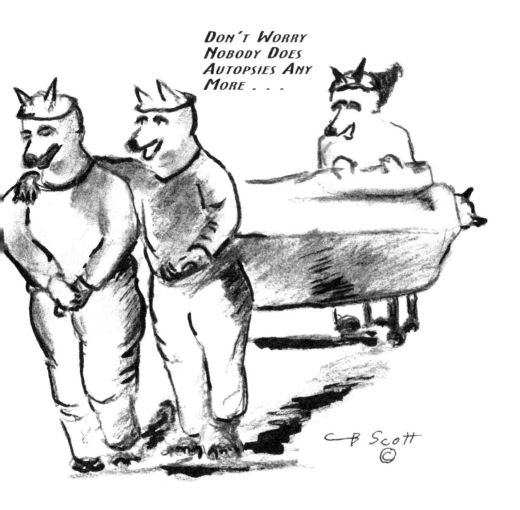

groups of doctors who were good doctors but "had no idea of how badly they had been doing before the measurement process began." Once they knew they had problems, they found what they were and fixed them.[21]

I can certainly see why reporting systems are popular with state legislatures. They are relatively cheap and less controversial than other ways to do something about the malpractice and medical errors problems. I have several reservations about them. First, raw numbers can be quite misleading. Referral centers, both academic teaching hospitals and the larger hospitals in a state like Wyoming, will tend to get the sicker cases because they have better resources to manage them. This may lead to poorer average results.

This phenomenon is well known, so risk adjustments are applied to the statistics, but that science can be imperfect and questions over it are likely to cause reported bad results to be ignored. In the New York case discussed earlier, the hospital thought their poor results were the result of inadequate risk adjustment until outside analysis showed differently. Second, particularly for individual doctors and smaller hospitals, the numbers of many kinds of cases are simply too small for statistically valid results.

Statistical bad luck can make a good doctor look bad and good luck can make a bad doctor look good. The third problem is that even if you make the reporting mandatory, an error reporting system will be defeated if the providers are motivated to bury their errors rather than finding them. An error not recognized can't be reported. In fact, a poorly designed system can make this problem worse — bad statistics can encourage lawsuits and can scare off potential customers.

My conclusion is that an error reporting system or results reporting system is potentially a part of an effective quality improvement effort. It may even be an essential part. However, I think it will be ineffective unless accompanied by 1) systematic analysis of the results to see if errors are being identified and then do something about them (the hospital in the New York example would have done nothing in the absence of outside analysis and follow up) and 2) changes in the system to remove incentives not to identify and report problems. This second requirement may apply only to systems designed explicitly to report errors; careful design of an outcomes based system may avoid this problem, but it will then require more analysis to identify problems.

A traditional means of quality control is a peer review process often going by the name of a mortality and morbidity review or conference. In this process, doctors periodically gather to review cases with bad outcomes to see what might be done differently next time. Atul Gawande in his delightful new book on modern surgical practice, <u>Complications, A Surgeon's Notes on an Imperfect Science</u>, has an excellent description of the weekly Morbidity and Mortality Conference in his hospital. All the surgeons, including the residents in training, are expected to attend. The chief residents report the problem cases. The assembled surgeons go over the case asking questions. Gawande describes the end of each discussion, "'What would you do differently?' a chairman asks concerning cases of avoidable harm. 'Nothing' is seldom an acceptable answer."[22]

The M & M Conference is a useful means of discovering and discussing errors with a view to preventing their future reoccurrence, but it has its shortcomings. For example, as Gawande describes it, it seems to have been restricted to surgeons. Health care is increasingly becoming a team endeavor. The other members of the team, the anesthesiologists and the nurses especially, can offer some different and very useful insights into problems. And there is the whole process leading up to the error.

As Gawande puts it so well, "The doctor is often only the final actor in a chain of events that set him or her up to fail. Error experts therefore believe that it's the process, not the individual in it, that requires closer examination and correction."[23]

In the M & M conferences, the participants are encouraged to be honest about what happened, and by and large they are. To encourage this, there is often a formal attempt to protect the participants by making the proceedings not discoverable in legal actions. Wyoming's law, for example is quite clear, "All reports, findings, proceedings and data of the professional standard review organizations is confidential and privileged, and is not subject to discovery or introduction into evidence in any civil action . . . ."[24]

However, the doctors do not fully trust that these protections would be adequate if a lawsuit occurred. At the January 26 meeting of the Wyoming Health Care Commission, Tom Lubnau, President of the Wyoming State Bar Association, was asked by a medical doctor on the commission if he knew whether peer review proceedings were discoverable in Wyoming. Mr. Lubnau's response was that he did not know how the Wyoming Supreme Court would rule on such a case.[25] In spite of the plain language in the law cited above, the annotations to that section of the published statutes report a case where the Supreme Court held that the trial court has an obligation to weigh the interests of the party seeking discovery against the patient's privacy interests.[26]

Having read the case, I think Mr. Lubnau's reaction was accurate; there are some other issues in the case so it is not at all clear how the Wyoming Supreme Court would rule on the issue in its pure form.

Both the question and the answer illustrate the fear of personal liability reaching even the time-honored effort of peer review. I don't know what we legislators can do to further protect the peer review process if the courts may ignore the protections we have already put in the law.

Gawande goes on to describe an effort over a number of years by the anesthesiologists to eliminate errors in their practice. In 1978 Jeffrey Cooper, an engineer, published a paper entitled "Preventable Anesthesia Mishaps: A Study of Human Factors." The paper found the most common errors were those relating to the patient's breathing. It listed the problems, often involving the anesthesia machine, that caused the errors. Gawande reports, "Just as important Cooper enumerated a list of contributory factors, including inadequate experience, inadequate familiarity with equipment, poor communications among team members, haste, inattention and fatigue."(27)

Cooper's paper generated interest and controversy among anesthesiologists and then in 1982 Dr. Ellison "Jeep" Pierce was elected vice president of the American Society of Anesthesiologists and was able to mobilize the society on the issue of errors. He teamed with Cooper and a whole series of fixes were developed for the problems.

Machines were redesigned with fallible humans in mind — on some anesthesia machines turning a dial clockwise increased the flow of oxygen and on others turning it counter clockwise did that, so dials were standardized. Locks were put in to prevent the accidental administration of more than one anesthesia gas at once. Some existing but frequently unused monitoring technology was made an official standard. The hours that anesthesia residents worked were shortened. It worked. In a decade the anesthesia death rate, which had varied during the 1960s to the 1980s from between one and two in every 10,000 operations, declined to one in every 200,000-plus operations. That was a twenty-fold decrease in what had been the source of 3,500 deaths a year.(28)

What was done for anesthesia is similar to what is being done in many other fields. The way the National Transportation Safety Board and the airline industry have analyzed air crashes to improve safety and prevent future accidents is an example everyone is aware of. The work of Edward W. Demming and the work at General Electric and others under the banner of Six Sigma are the same kind of efforts. Tom Lubnau, who I mentioned earlier, gave a presentation to the January meeting of the Wyoming Health Care Commission on the similar efforts in the firefighting community (he is a volunteer fireman as well as an attorney). He urged the commission to get a similar program adopted in health care.

Anesthesia is not the only medical success story of this kind — other parts of medicine have made similar efforts. I cited the institutional efforts of Johns Hopkins earlier. This kind of systematic identification of errors and fixing them remains, however, the exception rather than the rule. As I see it the task for policy makers is to reverse this and make it the rule.

As I discussed in the previous chapter, one of the obstacles is the fear of individual liability that the tort liability system engenders. I asked Dr. Brody, president of Johns Hopkins, how much of the problem he thought was caused by our tort liability system. He said 40 percent.[29] That strikes me as reasonable. The infallibility culture problem still looms large as does the normal human resistance to changes and the fact the sources of many errors are not obvious.

Brody and the anesthesiologists and others have shown how much can be done even in the presence of today's tort liability system. At the same time their efforts are not becoming universal and Johns Hopkins was able to act in part because it owns its own captive malpractice insurance company and can act against the advice of its lawyers. Many of the obstacles that confronted Johns Hopkins came from tradition, the medical culture, hierarchical customs, and the need for top management support, all independent of the tort system. My view is that to get a more universal error reduction effort, removing the tort liability obstacle is a necessary, but not sufficient step. The evidence also shows considerable success is possible, even given the tort liability obstacles.

So what should the state policy maker do? We have discussed a number of specific fixes of which I think the electronic medical record holds the most promise. I said earlier that the most promising approach is to change the system to one that puts patient safety first. I want to duplicate across the whole system what leaders like the anesthesiologists and Johns Hopkins have done for specific parts of it.

My proposal is the Health Care Errors Commission that I discussed in the previous chapter. It would replace the tort liability system and eliminate that personal fear. It would protect the peer review institution. Since we can't guarantee the courts will obey the laws protecting the confidentiality of peer review, fear of use of peer review proceedings in lawsuits is eroding the usefulness of that institution. Peer reviews plus commission reviews can crack the culture of personal infallibility without removing the healthy pressure for safe performance.

The errors commission can deal with the payment system incentives by denying providers compensation for fixing their errors, something that becomes possible because the commission's administrative proceedings will be quicker and cheaper than court proceedings. If properly staffed and managed, it would be a mechanism for doing the kind of studies Jeffrey Cooper did for anesthesia. It would operate much like the NTSB does for airline crashes. Moreover, as it produced successes, it should spark similar efforts by hospitals and other institutions and by provider groups.

My premise is that these groups want to eliminate errors and will be much happier practicing in a culture that puts patient safety first. They are frustrated that our present culture doesn't allow it, and they don't know how to get there. An errors commission can lead the way.

Chapter 3, Footnotes

(1) Kenneth I. Shine, 2001 Robert H. Ebert Memorial Lecture, "Health Care Quality and How to Achieve It," published by The Milbank Memorial Fund, 645 Madison Avenue, New York, NY, 2002.

(2) Lucian L. Leape, "Error in Medicine," Journal of the American Medical Association, Vol. 272, No. 23, December 21, 1994, page 1851.

(3) Leape, Ibid, page 1851.

(4) Shine, Ibid, page 1.

(5) Leape, Ibid, page 1852.

(6) Atul Gawande, Complications, A Surgeon's Notes on an Imperfect Science, Picador, Henry Holt and Company 2002, pages 62-63.

(7) National Conference of State Legislatures, "Medical Errors & System Safety: State Strategies Seek to Avoid 'Blame Game'"; State Health Notes, Vol. 24, No. 398, June 16, 2003, page 1.

(8) "Era of Errors," Health Care Purchaser, published by National Health Care Purchasing Institute, May 2000, pages 1 and 4.

(9) Health Care Purchaser, Ibid, p. 1.

(10) Aiken et al, "Hospital Nurse Staffing and Patient Mortality, Nurse Burnout, and Job Dissatisfaction," JAMA, October 23, 20??, Vol. 288, No. 16, pages 1987-1993.

(11) Shine, Ibid, p 5.

(12) Dr. John Brody, M.D., President, Johns Hopkins University, presentation to Wyoming Medical Center staff, Casper, Wyoming, December 19, 2003.

(13) Institute of Medicine, Crossing the Quality Chasm; A New Health System for the 21st Century, 2001, National Academy of Sciences, page 17. Note: this is in the advanced copy; the page in the final report might be slightly different.

(14) George C. Halvorson and George J. Isham, M.D., "Epidemic of Care," published by Jossey-Bass, a Wiley Imprint, 2003, page 27.

(15) Kim D. Slocum, "Rising Health Care Costs: Who's to Blame? What Can We Do?" Spectrum, Vol. 77, No. 3, Summer 2004, page 38 Spectrum is a publication of the Council of State Governments. Slocum cites J. Goldsmith et al., "Federal Health Information Policy: A Case of Arrested Development," Health Affairs, July/August 2003, as his authority.

(16) Dr. Molly Coye, M.D., William Bernstein, J.D., et al., policy monograph "Spending Our Money Wisely: Improving America's healthcare system by investing in healthcare information technology," Health Technology Center and Manatt, Phelps and Phillips, May 2003, page 12.

(17) Testimony of Dr. Paul Ellwood, Jackson Hole Group, before the Joint Interim Labor, Health and Social Services Committee, Wyoming Legislature, August 2003, author's recollection. See also Dr. Paul Ellwood, "Crossing the Health Policy Chasm, 'HEROIC Pathways,'" Jackson Hole Group, July 11, 2003.

(18) Shine, Ibid, p. 8.

(19) Mimi Marchev, Jill Rosenthal and Maureen Booth, "How States Report Medical Errors to the Public: Issues and Barriers," National Academy for State Health Policy, October 2003.

(20) National Conference of State Legislatures, State Health Notes, "Medical Errors & System Safety: State Strategies Seek to Avoid 'Blame Game'", State Health Notes, Vol. 24, No. 398, June 16, 2003, page 1.

(21) Halvorson and Isham, Ibid, page 29.

(22) Atul Gawande, Ibid, pages 58-62.

(23) Gawande, Ibid, page 64.

(24) W.S. 35-17-105.

(25) Personal observation by author, Wyoming Health Care Commission meeting, January 26, 2004.

(26) W.S. 35-17-105, annotations following text of statute, Wyoming Statutes Annotated, 2003 Edition, LexisNexis. Case cited is Harston v. Campbell County Memorial Hospital, 913 P. 2n 870 (Wyo. 1996).

(27) Gawande, Ibid, page 64.

(28) Gawande, Ibid, pages 64-69.

(29) Brody, Ibid.

Chapter 4

FAILURE TO IMPLEMENT PROVEN PRACTICES

A problem closely related to the problem of medical errors is the failure of medicine to implement many proven effective treatments and practices. This failure varies from slowness to adopt proven new practices to failure to follow some of medicines oldest science-based practices. A related problem we will discuss is how to identify the new practices that really are effective.

Some of the failures really should be classified as medical errors. For example the practice of careful hand washing and disinfection dates back to 1865 when Sir Joseph Lister realized that Pasteur's discoveries about bacteria had implications for surgical infections. This was a major advance; pre-Listerian surgery had up to a 50 percent mortality rate. Yet in 2003 when Johns Hopkins University Hospital set out to reduce its infection rate, one of the things it discovered was that some of its staff, including some of the senior attending physicians, had gotten sloppy about hand washing.[1] This is not lack of knowledge, it's the natural human tendency to cut corners and has to be classified as a medical error problem.

The IOM publication "Crossing the Quality Chasm" has a table entitled "Examples of Quality Health Care in the United States — Underuse: Did Patients Receive the Care They Should Have Received?"[2] The table is 40 pages long and lists various therapies and preventive measures that are well established and should be routinely received by everyone who meets the proper medical criteria. For example, the value of the use of drugs called beta blockers after heart attacks has been well established for more than 20 years. "Crossing the Quality Chasm" reports, "Beta blocker therapy can reduce post-MI [heart attack] mortality by as much as 25 percent, although beta blockers should not be given with certain conditions (e.g. low left ventricular ejection fraction, pulmonary edema)." It then lists five studies of the percentage of good

55

candidates who actually received beta blockers. The studies were published between 1995 and 1998 and showed a percentage receiving beta blockers that varied between 21 percent and 78 percent.[3]

On the same issue, Brody reported Johns Hopkins discovered that only 54 percent of its MI patients got appropriate beta blocker therapy on discharge and as of December 2003, was embarrassed that they had succeeded in raising that percentage only to 80 percent, a good percentage by contemporary American standards.[4] Halvorson and Isham report that 40 percent of Americans do not receive the beta blocker therapy when appropriate after heart attack, but report that their HMOs have achieved rates of 97 percent (Kaiser Permanente) and 98 percent (Health Partners).[5]

Diabetes care provides another set of similar examples. The American Diabetes Association (ADA) has developed an excellent, science-based set of standards for diabetes care. Halvorson and Isham report that two-thirds of America's doctors do not meet those standards.[6] Take one example. Diabetes can cause blindness as a result of damage from high blood sugar to the blood vessels in the retina of the eye. This blindness can be prevented by using lasers if the damage is spotted in time. I have Type 2 diabetes. My doctor both looks at my eyes himself and has insisted that I get a dilated eye exam from an ophthalmologist every year. The dilated eye exam is the standard. The IOM shows that in three studies from 1993 through 1995 only between 49 percent and 61 percent of appropriate diabetes patients met this standard.[7]

The current American medical system is inexcusably slow to implement many well proven therapies. Porter and Teisberg report, "It takes, on average, 17 years for the results of clinical trials to become standard clinical practice."[8] Again, well trained, well meaning people just are not getting the job done right. This is a system design problem that both health care professionals and health policy makers need to worry about.

Not all the failures in the IOM report are failures of the medical community. The general public must be held responsible for some, including the problems with childhood immunizations. The value of these immunizations is well proven.

There are well established professional organizations that set the recommendations for which immunizations are needed. The states in combination with the federal government have acted to make the vaccines readily available and affordable by everyone.

In Wyoming anyone can take a child to the local Public Health Office and get the vaccinations either cheap or free depending on their income, and this is typical. The states enforce vaccination as a mandatory condition of public school attendance. Many immunizations should be received well before school age, but we enforce at school age because we haven't identified a good way to comprehensively enforce it earlier.

The Wyoming law reads, "Any person attending, full or part time, any public or private school, kindergarten through twelfth grade shall within thirty (30) days of school entry, provide to the appropriate school official written documentary proof of immunization."[9] If the student doesn't have the immunizations (or, where a series over time is needed hasn't started them), the school administrator must exclude the student. The Legislature has changed the law a few times in recent years trying to improve the percentage that gets immunizations. In spite of this, our immunization percentage is poor.

The IOM citing the CDC in 1997 reports that only 74 percent of children 19-35 months of age had received all recommended childhood vaccinations.[10] The federal government's national immunization program reported that in 2001 the percentage of vaccination coverage in this same age group varied from a low of 63 percent in New Mexico to a high of 82 percent in Rhode Island, and 80 percent in Mississippi, Tennessee, Vermont, Virginia and Wisconsin. Most states were in the 70s. Wyoming was 74 percent.[11]

There are a few children who for medical reasons can't be vaccinated and all but two states permit a religious belief exemption. The numbers in these two categories are quite small. The main cause of the problem is parental apathy and ignorance and the influence of periodic anti-vaccine campaigns by assorted quacks, kooks and misguided conspiracy theorists. My observation is that much of the anti-vaccine agitation in this country comes from people on the extreme political right. By contrast, I'm told that in England it's often the loony left that's the source of the trouble.

Troubles with extremists over vaccinations are not confined to the developed world. In June 2004, The Economist reported that state authorities in the northern Nigerian state of Kano had suspended polio vaccination because the local imams were claiming polio vaccination was a Western plot to make Muslims sterile. The result was a resurgence of polio, which was then exported to 10 previously polio-free African countries.[12]

The low vaccination rate is dangerous. We get complacent because our vaccination rate has been high enough that we now avoid most of the childhood diseases, but we are skating down the edge of having enough unvaccinated kids to sustain an epidemic. These diseases can be very serious and they are still around. I personally had whooping cough (pertussis, the P of the DPT vaccine) as an adult (the childhood vaccine wears off with time) and I can understand how it could be fatal in a young child. I remember a diphtheria outbreak in Casper, Wyoming, in the late 1950s when I was in junior high. There were six cases and three of the children involved died.

One of the problems with medical adoption of new therapies and techniques is that not all of the new things that come out are beneficial. New drugs, even ones that have passed FDA scrutiny, sometimes have problems that show up only after prolonged usage.

Let me give a personal example. In 1997 the FDA approved a new diabetes drug named Rezulin.™ It was a new class of drug and it reduced insulin resistance at the cellular level. Since this is one of the problems with Type 2 diabetes, it was an important advance. I heard about it from various sources, including fellow diabetes patients. At one of my regular checkups, I asked my doctor. He said he thought it might be best to hold off on that one; he'd heard it might cause liver trouble. Sure enough, in 2000 the FDA took Rezulin™ off the market because it caused liver trouble too often. My doctor's conservatism was well justified. I point out there is a difference between a little conservatism on something like this and not adopting therapies like beta blockers years after careful trials have proved their value.

The Rezulin™ case is interesting because it raises another issue, the risk/benefit ratio. When the FDA acted, it had an easy decision. Other drugs had been developed and approved in 1999 (brand names Avandia,™ Actos™), which were in the same class and had similar benefits without the side effects.[13] If this had not happened, the FDA would have had a much tougher decision. Rezulin™ had significant benefits in controlling blood sugar in Type 2 diabetics. If there wasn't a better substitute available, would those benefits have out-weighed the risks? I suspect the answer may well have been yes, at least for some patients who could not achieve good control with the drugs available in other classes.

It may well be that with 20/20 hindsight both the FDA decision to allow Rezulin™ on the market when there was no substitute available and the decision to take it off after a substitute did become available were justified. I have never seen any careful analysis of this issue and would encourage somebody to do it — our policies on drug approvals could use some careful thought about risk benefit analysis. We need to apply different safety standards depending on the serious-ness of the disease being treated and the availability of alter-native treatments, and it appears the FDA does a poor job with this issue.

Another factor that justifies a degree of conservatism in adopting new approaches is that medicine is subject to fads just like most other forms of human endeavor. William Nolen in his delightful book A Surgeon's World recounts one of them, the gastric freeze. In the days before the role of the microorganism H. Pilori was discovered the duodenal ulcer was, in Nolen's words, "easy to treat but difficult to cure." Ten percent of the ulcer patient needed an operation which was a major one then carrying a mortality rate of between two and ten percent.

A group of surgeons got the idea that if they froze the patient's stomach, they could stop the flow of secretions that they believed caused the ulcers. They tried it in dogs and it worked. They tried it in humans. It worked, at least ini-tially. They published in both a professional journal (JAMA, May 12, 1962) and in the popular press ("They're Freezing Ulcers to Death," Readers Digest, January 1963). Patients read the Readers Digest and ran to their doctors.

Some resisted, some bought gastric freeze machines and proceeded. Nolen reports the results, "It wasn't long before the fears of the skeptics were confirmed. Six months after having their stomach frozen, it was learned most of the victims had their ulcers back." And there were complications that killed a few patients.

Nolen further reports, "It took a while for the news to get around — remember "breakthroughs always make the front page, failures show up in the obituary columns — but eventually it did . . . The entire episode, from the first 'freeze' to the last took about five years."[14] The gastric freeze is ancient enough history that most surgeons in practice today probably never heard of it, but Nolen's advice, "The next time you read of some miraculous medical innovation, some 'cure' for a previously incurable disease, some wonderful 'breakthrough,' think twice before you believe it . . ." is still valid today.[15]

So how are the good innovations that ought to be routinely adopted to be separated from the fads that are ineffective or even dangerous? This is where evidence-based medicine comes in.

The basic idea of evidence-based medicine is simple — get scientific evidence of which procedure or medicine works or which works best and base treatments on that evidence. Implementing that simple concept can be complicated and difficult.

Scientific evidence can be misunderstood, the studies can have unintended biases, the numbers involved can be too small to be statistically reliable, the studies can be too short and miss long-term effects — there are scores of things that can go wrong. An example was provided by the practice of autologous bone marrow transplants for advanced breast cancer. The procedure works for some other kinds of cancer. There was a study that suggested it might work for advanced breast cancer. That was evidence, but it wasn't adequate evidence.

It turned out that the study had a bias problem; the treated group was healthier to start with than the control group. With 20/20 hindsight, it's fair to say that the researchers, advocates and patients involved jumped to conclusions because they were desperate for something that worked reliably. The insurers objected to paying for the expensive treatments on the grounds they were experimental and unproven.

That led to a dispute that got into the political arena. A number of legislatures (not including Wyoming) yielded to temptation and got into the practice of medicine by mandating coverage for the procedure.

Then there were some large scale follow-up studies that showed the procedure did more harm than good.[16] The practice has been largely abandoned, but some researchers feel that it may be of benefit to some women and are trying to identify which ones. At this writing, the final answer on that issue must be regarded as unresolved, although the general use of the procedure has been discredited.

Be wary of claims that use of some procedure or pill is "evidence based." In much of the health policy world, "evidence-based medicine" has, for good reason, become one of the mantras. The result is that advocates and activists have taken to describing their favorite solutions as "evidence based" when in fact their evidence may be inadequate or just plain wrong.

Following the advice of recognized experts also should not be confused with evidence-based medicine. The advice of experts is quite useful when it is based on careful evaluation of scientific evidence and clinical experience. When, however, it is based on tradition, prejudice or theoretical reasoning not scientifically tested, it can be spectacularly wrong. A good expert should be right most of the time, but given the complexities of human biology most of the time is different from all the time.

Dr. Spock provides an example. His famous book, <u>Baby and Child Care</u>, is in general a fountain of common sense and sound advice. It was successfully used by two generations of parents as a guide. However, on one issue, Spock was very wrong. On the issue of whether to put babies to sleep on their stomachs or their backs, he cites two disadvantages of the back position: "If they vomit, they are more likely to choke on the vomitus. Also, they tend to keep the head turned toward the same side . . . This may flatten that side of the head." Then he advises, "I think it is preferable to accustom babies to sleeping on the stomach from the start if they are willing."[17] Subsequently, some careful research showed that putting babies to sleep on their stomachs contributes to the risk of Sudden Infant Death Syndrome (SIDS) and the evidence-based advice now is to put them to sleep on their backs.

The point is not that Spock was bad — when he wrote, the research had not been done yet — but that the advice of experts should not be confused with scientific evidence. In the absence of evidence, even the experts can be wrong.

The gold standard in evidence is the randomized controlled trial (RCT). A group of patients with similar problems or risk factors is obtained. One group is given the treatment being tested; another, the control group, is given a placebo or conventional therapy. The patients are assigned to one group or the other at random. If it's possible and safe, the patients and even their doctors don't know whether they are the treated group or the control group. The results are then compared to see what difference, if any, the treatments made.

There are some requirements for successful RCTs. The number of patients in each category has to be large enough for the results to be statistically valid. Biases in assignment of the patients to the control group or the treated group have to be avoided. If one group has more of some risk factor like smoking or is older, the results can be biased. Randomization is the principal means of preventing bias, but other sampling techniques also are used.

For example, if smoking is a risk factor as it often is, the researchers can separate the patients into smokers and non-smokers and randomly pick within each group so the control group and the treated group each have the same percentage of smokers. It is also often possible to make statistical adjustments for differences in risk factors in the two groups. A frequent problem can be a severity difference in the groups of patients being tested; this can be difficult to identify and adjust for.

Other factors can bias studies as well. As this is written in 2004, there is a dispute over the value of a new technique, the virtual colonoscopy. Colonoscopies are recommended for people over 50 for early detection of colorectal cancer, a disease that is all too common and a major killer. For both men and women, it is the third most common cause of cancer death (after lung and prostate or breast cancer). The odds of successful treatment are much better if the disease is detected early and the colonoscopy is the way to detect it early. In a regular colonoscopy, a doctor inserts a scope into the rectum and looks for cancers and polyps that may develop into cancers. The procedure is very unpleasant and not free of risk, so many people avoid it.

The virtual colonoscopy uses scans from the outside, which are not unpleasant for the patient. The scans carry some radiation risk particularly where CT scans are used. I have not seen an evaluation of the degree of risk. Such an evaluation is needed to make sure the risks of the scans involved do not exceed their benefits.

If virtual colonoscopies are accurate, they could save a lot of lives because more people will be willing to undergo them. The Wall Street Journal published a news story covering a dispute as to whether they do work. The New England Journal of Medicine (NEJM) published an article saying the new virtual scans were just as good as the traditional colonoscopy and the Journal of the American Medical Association (JAMA) published one saying the virtual scans missed between half and two thirds of the potentially cancerous polyps. The partisans of the NEJM article says the JAMA study used an outdated technique while the JAMA partisans say their study is relevant because it uses the techniques and training currently available to most patients.[18]

I suspect that it is possible that the design of one or both studies was influenced by economic and guild/jurisdictional factors — gastroenterologists do traditional colonoscopies, but radiologists do virtual ones. I think we're in for a scientific debate with competing studies for a while. Eventually the evidence on one side or the other may be convincing, or it may come down to a matter of consumer preference. There could well be an accuracy vs. comfort vs. risk of the procedure trade-off where going either way could make sense. I also think one comment The Wall Street Journal reporter made in the story is right on point: "So who's right? The answer offers a telling lesson into the limitations of scientific research and medical politics. And it should serve as a warning to doctors and patients against placing too much stock in any single medical study."

RCTs are very common. In the United States the Food and Drug Administration (FDA) normally requires an RCT comparing the new drug with a placebo before it will approve a new drug. RCTs often are used in evaluating other issues including new medical devices and new test and treatments. The numbers are astounding. As of 2003 the Cochrane Register of Controlled Trials included 360,000 studies out of an estimated one million published randomized trials.[19]

In addition to the simple volume of trials, the articles describing the trials are slow going for anyone, doctor or layman, reading them. There are always issues about the validity of the trials. The methodology for selecting the sample, administering the treatment, and evaluating the results has to be described in detail because the methodology can change the results. There are always issues about potential biases in all these aspects of the trials. Often the patients participating in the trial were recruited to have certain characteristics and there is a question as to whether the results apply to other patients. The net effect of the volume of material and the difficulty in understanding it is that it is a practical impossibility for any doctor to be aware of all the science available even in a relatively narrow area of medicine.

In answer to this problem, the Cochrane Collaboration that maintains the registry is conducting systematic reviews of the trials in different areas. The Cochrane Collaboration is a network of scientific volunteers who conduct systematic reviews of medically related trials using standard protocols. It traces its roots to activities started in Oxford, England, in the 1970s with the first Cochrane center established in England in 1992 and funded by the British National Health Service. It now is a loose network of 14 centers, independently grant funded, which coordinates the activities of the volunteer scientists.[20]

The purpose of the Cochrane reviews is to make the net results of the large number of RCTs usable by the medical community. The reviews analyze the strengths and limitations of each study and try to integrate the results to reach summary conclusions on the current state of knowledge. Again the numbers are large. As of 2003, the collaboration had issued 1,600 reviews and had 1,200 underway of an estimated 10,000 needed.[21] As of 2004, the number of reviews done was approaching 4,000. And reviews have to be periodically redone as new studies are completed. Assuming some reasonable priority setting in the reviews done, the percentage of the needed areas covered is probably much higher than these raw numbers indicate, but still the task is daunting and the individual physician still will have difficulty keeping up in his or her own area of specialty.

The Internet is a big help in this area. The Cochrane Collaboration is online and subscriptions are available for a fee that is quite affordable for an institution like a hospital. Some states are moving to make it available to all their citizens. In Wyoming the State Library has purchased access and any Wyoming citizen can get access from his home computer through the library. My observation of the various online sources, both Cochrane and others, is that they take time to sift through and find what you need. Time is something in short supply for many of us, especially a busy doctor. One of my objectives as a member of the Advisory Board of the United States Cochrane Center is to try to get the Cochrane materials quicker and easier for the busy doctor to find and use.

The Cochrane reviews are something that an individual patient with a disease might want to look at. I have done so myself. Like articles describing RCTs, they are slow going and there are some things in them you may have to ask a knowledgeable friend or relative about to understand, but an educated layman can make sense out of the results. You may even find some things that will educate your doctor. With the size of the knowledge base available, remember that it is unreasonable to expect your doctor to be completely aware of all the science on any issue.

Remember that you and your disease are only a small part of your doctor's practice, but 100 percent of yours. You can afford to spend more time digging out information on your problem than he can. Having said that, your doctor has a professional knowledge of the underlying science and a bank of clinical experience that the layman can't match. Pay attention if he says, "I don't think that research applies to your case because . . ."

Another problem with the RCTs is that in spite of the number of trials that have been done, there are often no trials that precisely answer a particular medical question. For example, drug trials often are done against a placebo not a competing brand name drug of the same class. You can compare the two drugs by comparing how they each did against placebos, but often there are enough differences in the trials to make the results of that comparison unclear.

Again, you have to fall back on the professional judgment of your doctor, and sometimes he will have to do a little experimenting to see what works for you. This may be true even where an RCT provides an answer. If a trial shows drug A is better than drug B for 80 percent of the patients, it is still possible you will be in the 20 percent for whom drug B is the better choice.

Sometimes, things work the other way. A study will suggest conclusions beyond what it actually shows, and with a little common sense those conclusions still can be useful. For example, a major study was done showing that tight control of blood sugars leads to a greatly reduced probability of complications for diabetics. The study was done using just Type 1 (formerly called juvenile) diabetes, so strictly speaking it doesn't apply to Type 2 (formerly known as adult onset) diabetes, which is a different disease with different causes. However, for both diseases it is the high blood sugar that causes many of the complications so it's reasonable to assume that tight control will improve the results for Type 2 diabetics as well.

Randomized Controlled Trials are not the only useful source of scientific medical evidence. Epidemiological studies where populations are followed over time and results are linked to various characteristics or behaviors are very useful — they can produce knowledge that is unavailable any other way. There are various other studies that can be useful.

The practical problem for even the best doctor remains keeping up with the sheer volume of knowledge. They come out of medical school and post-graduate training (residency) with a relatively up-to-date knowledge base, but it is imperfect and gets rapidly out of date. I have heard some health policy experts say that doctors are forever frozen into the practices they learned in medical school. This is unjust to the vast majority of doctors, but it has an element of truth. Because of the size of the body of new evidence, every doctor will from time to time fall back on tradition and what he learned in medical school.

Every good doctor makes an effort to keep up. Their techniques are varied. They read professional journals. They go to professional presentations at meetings and conventions and talk to fellow doctors. Those that are comfortable with modern computer technology will use the Internet to access the Cochrane Collaboration or the collection of the National Library of Medicine at the NIH. They associate with medical schools or residency programs and stay current by clinical teaching. In Wyoming, if I find a doctor who is teaching WWAMI medical students on clinical rotation, I will suspect that the interchange with the students and the need to teach is keeping that doctor up to date.[22]

The health policy problem is that none of these techniques is perfect because the possible knowledge base is too large. I think berating the doctors to do a better job in keeping up or even legislating continuing education is likely to be ineffective. Continuing education can be useful, but the volume of new knowledge is too large for continuing education. Also, it is all together too easy to market a continuing education course where the doctor learns more about his golf swing than medicine. The challenge for health policy is to engineer the health care system to maximize the use of evidence-based medicine.

One innovation I would like to see more of is the development of practice guidelines for specific diseases and circumstances. These are developed by getting knowledgeable experts together to review the best evidence available and hammer out guidelines for how to manage specific diseases or symptoms. The results are just guidelines. A doctor still has to use professional judgment to make sure the patient fits the guidelines. Making sure the patient's diagnosis is right and evaluating other conditions the patient may have to see if departures from the guidelines are warranted both require use of the doctor's clinical knowledge and experience. For example Bell's Palsy, a partial paralysis of various facial muscles, can be quite disabling for anyone unfortunate enough to get it. It often resolves on its own with time, but not always. The drugs that treat it raise blood sugar, a problem for anyone with diabetes. A doctor with a patient with both problems has to use some judgment. With that said, the guidelines can be very useful in ensuring that patients get scientifically valid treatment.

A good source of practice guidelines should be associations formed to fight specific diseases. I already have mentioned the guidelines that the American Diabetes

Association has put together for that disease; they are very highly regarded.[23] Other associations should be encouraged to undertake similar efforts. Maine tried developing guidelines locally and used them to shield practitioners from malpractice liability, but their efforts appear to have fallen into disuse. I suspect, but cannot prove, they were ineffective as protections against lawsuits.

Managed care at its best also can be a source of translating evidence-based medicine into practice. It can coerce practitioners into using scientifically based practices. The doctors sometimes don't like the process and criticize it as cookbook medicine, but if the practices being enforced were carefully chosen by professional evaluation of the scientific evidence available, it can work very well. Recall the highest rates of beta blocker usage I cited earlier. They were achieved by HMOs.

The basic problem remains, however. Medicine is too slow to implement proven practices and the process is too uneven with too many patients denied the benefits of advances. This points to the same lack of an adequate quality control process that I discussed in the chapter on Medical Errors. I think the same remedy — a Medical Errors Commission willing to use and enforce the results of careful systems analysis is indicated.

Chapter 4, Footnotes

(1) Dr. John Brody, M.D., President, Johns Hopkins University, presentation to Wyoming Medical Center staff, Casper, Wyoming, December 19, 2003.

(2) Institute of Medicine, National Academy of Sciences, Crossing the Quality Chasm, National Academy Press, Washington, D.C., 2001, pages 264-304.

(3) IOM, Ibid, pages 301-302.

(4) Brody, Ibid.

(5) George C. Halvorson and George J. Isham, M.D., "Epidemic of Care," pages 16, 17 and 170.

(6) Halvorson & Isham, Ibid, page 160.

(7) IOM, Ibid, pages 279-280.

(8) Michael E. Porter and Elizabeth Olmstead Teisberg, "Redefining Competition in Health Care, Harvard Business Review, June 2004, page 65.

(9) W.S. (Wyoming Statute) 21-4-309(a).

(10) IOM, Ibid, page 264.

(11) National Immunization Program, fact sheet distributed by the CDC, citing the National Immunization Survey.

(12) The Economist, "A Virus Revives," June 26, 2004, page 52.

(13) The Diabetes Advisor, Diabetes Forecast, June 2004, page 25. Rezulin^{TM} is the brand name for troglitazone. Avandia is the brand name for rosiglitazone. Actos is the brand name for pioglitazone. Both Avandia and Actos have side effects too, but they are rarer and easier to treat.

(14) William A. Nolen, M.D., A Surgeon's World, Fawcett, 1970, pages 235-238.

(15) Nolen, Ibid, pages 241-242.

(16) Halvorson & Isham, Ibid, pages 58-59.

(17) Dr. Benjamin Spock, Baby and Child Care, Pocket Books, Simon & Schuster, copyright 1945, 1946, 1957, 1968 & 1976, page 199.

(18) Tara Parker-Pope, "A Tale of Two Studies: Cutting Through the Confusion on Virtual Colonoscopies," The Wall Street Journal, April 27, 2004, page D1.

(19) Alicia Ault, "Climbing a Medical Everest," Science, Vol. 300, June 27, 2003, pages 2024 and 2025.

(20) For a more complete description of the Cochrane Collaboration and randomized trials, see either the Ault article in Science cited above or Kay Dickerson and Drummond Renie, "Registering Clinical Trials," Journal of the American Medical Association (JAMA), July 23/30, 2003, Vol. 290 No.4, pages 516-518.

(21) Ault, Ibid, page 2024.

(22) WWAMI is the rural medical school program of the University of Washington Medical School that serves as the medical school for rural Washington and the states of Wyoming, Alaska, Montana and Idaho. Its third- and fourth-year students do clinical rotations with practicing doctors in all these states.

(23) See Halvorson and Isham, op. cit. pages 22 and 160-163.

Chapter 5

UNNECESSARY MEDICAL EXPENDITURES

"Work expands so as to fill the time available for its completion."
— Parkinson's Law, C. Northcote Parkinson[1]

The United States is widely reported to have a problem with expenditures for medically unnecessary care. A front-page article in the Wall Street Journal in December 2003 reported an estimate that our country could cut its annual health care expenditures by 15-30 percent by operating more efficiently and reducing medical error.[2] The same article reported that David Wennberg of the Center for Outcomes Research and Evaluation at the Maine Medical Center reported that Medicare could trim 30 percent of its budget by bringing the highest spending regions of the U.S. in line with the lowest spending ones.

In his book, The Brave New World of Health Care, Richard Lamm reports on our overuse of X-rays and then claims, "Similarly it is estimated that 40 percent of our lab work is simply unnecessary . . . ."[3] In August 2004, The Wall Street Journal, citing findings published in the Annals of Internal Medicine, reported on overuse of follow-up colonoscopies costing $1,600 each on patients who had benign polyps and other abnormalities removed from their colons.[4]

Spending for unnecessary medical care is not a new problem. In 1991 a legislative committee I chaired held a hearing on rising health care costs and published a report which said, "The Health Insurance Association of America representative estimated that about 20 percent of the premium cost goes for unnecessary medical care. Various sources have stated that as much as 30 percent to 50 percent of specific surgeries are unnecessary. The Wyoming Trial Lawyers Association notes that according to one study, as much as 11 percent of medical procedures doctors perform on patients is unnecessary."[5]

A key study in this area was done by Drs. Elliott Fisher and David Wennberg and their associates and published in February 2003 as a pair of articles in the Annals of Internal Medicine, the professional journal of the American College of Physicians-American Society of Internal Medicine.[6] The study covered Medicare beneficiaries hospitalized between 1993 and 1995 for hip fracture, colorectal cancer and myocardial infarction (heart attack) and a representative sample from the Medicare Current Beneficiary Survey (1992-1995).

The study controlled for differences among regions in prices of services and health status of the patients studied. The study found ". . . patients in higher spending regions received approximately 60 percent more care. The increased utilization was explained by more frequent physician visits, especially in the inpatient setting . . . more frequent tests and minor (but not major) procedures, and increased use of specialists and hospitals."[7] It is important to note that the higher spending regions refers not to regions with higher prices or reimbursements, but ones with more utilization of services for a given amount of illness.

Part 2 of their articles concluded, "Medicare enrollees in higher-spending regions receive more care than those in lower-spending regions but do not have better health outcomes or satisfaction with care."[8]

Fisher found the differences in minor rather than major services. Part 2 of the articles says, "The additional utilization in high-spending regions is largely devoted to discretionary services that have previously been demonstrated to be associated with the local supply of physicians and hospital resources."[9] This is a specialized application of Parkinson's general law quoted at the start of this chapter. The resources are there so the work expands to use them.

The Fisher study found no variation in the rate of major surgeries among the regions. This finding suggests that any differences in the medical community about the circumstances in which patients really need major surgeries are based on differences in professional opinions and are not the result of local circumstances, particularly economic circumstances. This does not rule out a rate of unnecessary major surgeries which is constant among the regions studied.

Indeed, a number of sources suggest the U.S. has an important rate of unnecessary major procedures. The Commonwealth Fund published a chart in its 2002 Chartbook showing a high rate of inappropriate or questionable use of a number of procedures including hysterectomies (16 percent inappropriate, 25 percent questionable for a 41 percent total).[10] Synthesizing a number of professional studies relating to the treatment of heart attacks in the U.S. and Canada, David Cutler finds evidence that the United States over-utilizes two major procedures, bypass surgery and angioplasty. He reports, ". . . a typical heart attack patient is many times more likely to get bypass surgery or angioplasty in the United States than Canada. Any yet, survival after a heart attack is virtually identical in the two countries. Not everyone in the United States needs such intensive care."[11] The Commonwealth Fund's chart puts the rate of inappropriate and questionable use of bypass surgery and angioplasty at 44 percent and 42 percent, respectively.[12]

Bluntly speaking, where there is a surplus of doctors and hospitals, they make work for themselves. This is expensive for Medicare or whoever is paying the bills and on average does the patients no good and may even be slightly harmful.

Remember Dr. Wennberg's conclusion cited at the outset of the chapter that Medicare could reduce its spending 30 percent by reducing the spending to the levels found in the lower cost regions. His data relate only to the Medicare population, but there is no reason to think the results would be different for the rest of the population. The suggestion then is that we could reduce our total health care expenditures by 30 percent by eliminating unnecessary care without doing any harm to our health. Thirty percent would go a long way toward explaining the differences between the United States and the rest of the developed world.

There is another source of unnecessary medical care, defensive medicine, related to our tort liability system. Our tort system is similar enough across the whole country that we should expect to see a level of defensive medicine in every region. The Fisher study looked at regional differences so a minimum level of unnecessary medical care to protect providers from the tort system would have been a constant and not identified by that study. There is one study showing some (6-10 percent) state by state differences in defensive medicine depending on whether or not the state has enacted the MICRA reforms.[13] If more of the higher spending regions also lacked MICRA, then some of the unnecessary care the Fisher study found could have been caused by defensive medicine, but that is not clear from the published articles.

My view is that the unnecessary medical care probably has multiple causes. For example, a surgeon I know has told me of seminars where the makers on the newest medical devices ply the doctors with horror stories of patients whose problems were missed because their new device wasn't used. Mix the doctors' natural desire to do the best possible job for their patients with the fear of being sued if they leave any stone unturned. Then add whatever additional personal earnings they may get from reading the test, and you have quite a recipe for selling new and expensive medical technology.

Sometimes the doctor's desire to do the best possible job for his or her patients can be distorted by his experience. I once had a personal experience illustrating this. Thirty years ago when I was working in Washington, D.C., I went for a checkup at the health plan I was enrolled in. In the absence of any symptoms, the doctor wanted me to have a chest X-ray to catch any lung cancer that might have started. This was a staff model HMO, so neither the doctor nor the HMO got any extra compensation for an X-ray.

Taking a chest X-ray for a male in his 20s who had never used tobacco is well beyond the normal standard of care, so I don't see how fear of tort liability could have motivated the recommendation. I turned the recommendation down on the grounds that the risk of the radiation involved was greater than the chance it would do me any good. I questioned the doctor as to why he wanted it done. It turned out he had just lost a friend to lung cancer who was a young non-smoker. That is exceedingly rare and even if it happened, the chance that an X-ray would catch the cancer in a stage where successful treatment would be possible was and is very low. It was the doctor's unusual personal experience that was influencing his view of what he ought to do for his patients. Doctors are human, and personal experience can override statistics on what is necessary.

How much is unnecessary medical care costing us? As discussed in the previous chapter on Medical Malpractice, good statistics on the amount of defensive medicine are not available. I have seen estimates from 10 percent of total health care costs to 20 percent or more. If we add the 30 percent estimate based on the Fisher study to this range of estimates of defensive medicine, we get a range of between 40 percent and 50 percent of all U.S. health care expenditures being for medically unnecessary treatments.

My judgment is that this is too high, and there is at least partial overlap between the unnecessary care Fisher found and defensive medicine. Even if we cut the high end of the range in half and estimate 25 percent as being the medically unnecessary expenditure, we could get rid of if we were as efficient as the rest of the developed world. We could cut our total health care expenditures to 11 percent of GNP, close to the upper range of what is seen elsewhere.

This theory that unnecessary care is a major cause of the difference between the cost of health care in the United States and the rest of the developed world rests both our level of unnecessary care and the theory the other countries have avoided that. We have just discussed the best evidence I can find on our level of unnecessary care. What evidence I have seen for the rest of the developed world suggests it has some problems with unnecessary care, but nothing that approaches ours. For example, Lamm reports that in Great Britain the Royal College of Radiologists estimated that 20 percent of the X-rays taken were unnecessary, this at a time Great Britain used less than half the X-rays per capita used in the United States.[14]

For two reasons the rest of the world should have mostly avoided our unnecessary care problem. First, no where else has the legal system been allowed to run amok the way it does here; the rest of the world doesn't have a problem with malpractice that comes anywhere close to ours. Second, the rest of the world has either a government provided single-payer system or a universal care system closely regulated by the government. These systems prevent unneeded care with various degrees of success.

In 2001, The Wall Street Journal published comparisons of various national developed world systems as part of a special section on health care.[15] It divided the world into tax-based systems (e.g. Canada, U.K.), social insurance systems (e.g. Germany, France, Japan), and private insurance (U.S. and Switzerland, only). In the tax-based systems, government budgets are explicitly used to ration care to hold down costs, the degree of rationing depends on the willingness of the people to pay taxes. I think in the process of rationing the needed care, this system gets rid of the unneeded care.

In the social insurance systems there are very closely regulated quasi-public insurance carriers that provide a universal coverage. In general the tax-based systems are the cheapest, although their costs overlap those of the social insurance systems. The cheapest were the tax-based U.K. and Spanish systems at 6.7 percent and 7.1 percent of GNP, respectively. However the most expensive tax based system, Canada at 9.5 percent of GNP was more expensive than the cheapest social insurance systems, Japan at 7.6 percent and Austria at 8.2 percent, but cheaper than the top social insurance systems, Germany at 10.6 percent and France at 9.6 percent.

No one came close to our costs then at 13.6 percent of GNP although the only other private insurance system, Switzerland, came in second at 10.6 percent, tied with Germany. The Wall Street Journal reported the social insurance systems had some of our unnecessary care problems. "Moreover, there's a financial incentive for doctors to heap on care: Insurance carriers pay doctors on a fee-for-service basis. The more they do, the more they earn," and "The biggest complaint about social insurance systems is profligacy. Some critics charge that social insurance systems 'overtreat' their patients with more medicines and longer hospital stays."[16]

The Wall Street Journal accounts for the differences between our system and the social insurance systems as being due to higher doctors' earnings here and our massive administrative bureaucracy. As discussed in a subsequent chapter, prescription drugs are more expensive here. These are all differences, but the most important difference is other countries are holding down the unneeded care, by avoiding defensive medicine, regulating the high tech devices and rationing care through government budgets. This hypothesis needs a more thorough quantitative analysis, but I am convinced such an analysis will show unneeded care will be the most important factor driving up U.S. costs.

As we discussed in the previous chapter, some defensive medicine carries some risk for the patient, from the risks of both invasive procedures and ionizing radiation. There is evidence of this risk for other unnecessary care in the Fisher data, but the evidence is not very strong. They found that for acute heart attacks, the higher spending regions had a higher one-year mortality rate. The opposite was true, but to a lesser degree for hip fractures. I would speculate that the heart attack group showed more risk than the hip fractures because there are more "minor" but risky invasive procedures that can be done for that diagnosis than for hip fractures. Overall, Fisher said, "Observed mortality tended to be lower than predicted in the lowest [utilization] quintile [of regions] and equal to or higher than predicted in the highest quintile."[17]

Fisher and his colleagues did not measure the full extent of the harm that was done by unnecessary medical procedures. They were looking at the Medicare population and they were looking only at 30-day and one-year survival rates. These should have picked up most risks from invasive procedures, but in general would not have picked up risks from ionizing radiation, which leads to cancers that typically take longer than one year to develop. It is also riskier in a younger population that has more life span left in which to develop a cancer.

Having made the case that unnecessary medical care is a cause of excessive health care spending in the United States, let me express a couple of cautions. First, as will be discussed in a later chapter, administrative costs are higher in the U.S. than elsewhere and many experts believe that higher prices for procedures rather than the quantity of procedures performed explains the difference between the United States and the rest of the developed world. Second, in Wyoming we have fewer physicians per 100,000 population than almost every other state; we rank 47th. With some local exceptions, we don't have the physician surpluses that would lead to economically motivated unnecessary medical care, yet our health care costs are higher than most of the rest of the United States.

For example, Dr. David Crowder, M.D., working on reducing health costs for the coal industry, reported that Gillette,

Wyoming, had significantly higher per employee health costs than any of four other sites where one coal company did business. The differences ranged from about 25 percent to over 100 percent with the lowest costs being an area with high managed care penetration.[18] There are reasons for this including, discrimination against Wyoming by the Medicare program, lack of managed care, local hospital or other facility surpluses and lack of tort reform leading to higher malpractice insurance costs and increased defensive medicine. Still, our Wyoming experience suggests that economically motivated unnecessary care is, at most, one cause among many of American higher health care costs.

Solutions to our problem of unnecessary care are complex because its causes are complex. We need more well done research on the subject, but those of us in state legislatures have to act now on the basis of what is known.

The previous chapter on the tort liability system discussed the solution to the defensive medicine part of the equation. Later in this book as we examine solutions to our health care problems, how well the unnecessary care problem is dealt with will be one of the tests for evaluating the solutions.

Getting doctors and other providers good information on what care is needed and effective is a problem state legislatures can help with. As discussed in the previous chapter there are thousands of randomized control trials that provide useful information. The Cochrane Collaboration provides reviews of these trials that evaluate their strengths and weaknesses and summarize the current state of knowledge on many issues. Making this data base widely available within the state would be a cheap first step for a legislature to take.

Another step would be to charge a group of systems analysis and health care professionals with examining the most important tests and procedures, which are suspected of being defensive medicine. The most important could be selected either on dollar volume or risk to the patient. If such a group can come up with a set of practice guidelines on when to use and when not to use such tests and procedures, we then can start to reduce their unnecessary usage. This would be a task for the Medical Errors Commission proposed in previous chapters, but other organizations could do it as well.

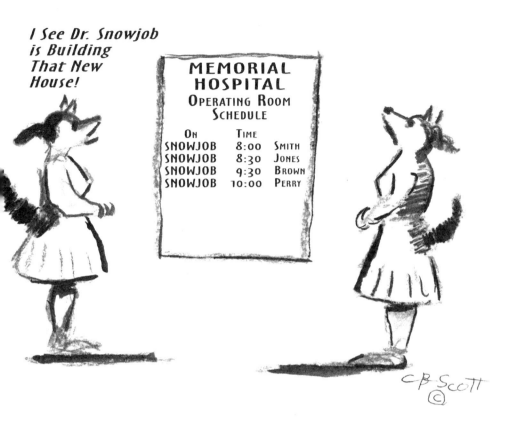

Other efforts have been made to reduce the growth in unnecessary expenditures by restricting the supply particularly of institutions. Certificate of Need (CON) where a health care institution had to show a need for services before it could be built or expanded was widely tried because it was a federal requirement for a time. The federal requirement went away and most states have in the past 15 or so years repealed their CON requirements on the grounds that they cost more in administration for both the governments and the institutions than they saved.

We in Wyoming repealed the general provision in 1987,[19] but have kept a degree of restriction on nursing home expansion. I remember talk in the Natrona County legislative delegation that the CON process was discriminating against our community, which illustrates one of the general problems CON had — all facilities are an important part of some legislator's district and political pressures promptly got involved.

HMOs also can be effective in reducing unnecessary care. I would speculate that staff model HMOs are more effective than ones that largely contract with private providers for services. In the latter case, depending on the nature of the contract, the providers can have some or all of the incentives for unnecessary care present in the fee for service system. The HMOs have tried various devices to cut down on unnecessary care, but they have found it difficult to discriminate administratively between reducing unnecessary care and rationing needed care.

In the process, they offended both providers and their customers resulting in political regulation and marketplace difficulties. Some of their efforts, like cutting short hospital maternity stays and giving doctors bonuses for keeping care down, were seized on by their opponents and used to beat them in the political arena. These problems are discussed along with the HMO efforts to use competition to hold down provider prices in Chapter 8 entitled "Competition in Health Care."

Currently disease management is one of the fads in health policy. Disease management covers a wide range of practices, but typically someone who's not a regular caregiver for the patient, often a nurse, follows up with the patient and the patient's caregivers to make sure proper protocols are actually followed. For a while my insurance company had a nurse who was calling me to make sure I got the proper diabetes care. I'm afraid that what she learned with me was that a working rancher does not stay near a telephone very long in daylight hours, and she had little effect on the care I got.

A major focus of disease management is to make sure that people with serious diseases get the preventive care they need. For example, disease management can include strategies to make sure people with high blood pressure take their medicine, or to make sure diabetics get regular A1c tests for high blood sugar and follow up with corrective action when the results are bad. However, an important component of disease management is to cut costs by cutting out pills, tests and procedures that the patient really doesn't need. I call disease management a fad, but there are instances where it pays. There also have been cases where it cost more than it saved. It appears to be a useful tool when used properly in the correct circumstances, and we don't yet fully understand how to use it properly and what are the correct circumstances.

End of life care is frequently cited in health policy circles as being excessive and involving much medically unnecessary care. A surprising percentage of a person's lifetime medical expenses can come in the last few months of life. The policy argument is that these costs don't do any good; the patient has a disease which kills him in spite of all medical science can do, so the expensive efforts were unnecessary. The counter argument is that we generally can't tell for sure what will happen so the care is justified because it may prolong the patient's life, and anyway someone sick enough so they die is sick enough to need expensive care. The truth is somewhere in between.

For some conditions, death is inevitable and the treatments to delay it cause significant disability. For example, chemotherapy for cancer basically works by killing the cancer cells slightly faster than the patient. For some types of cancers, it beats the cancer back and prolongs life, but at quite a cost in unpleasant side effects for the patients. I recently had a friend who died of colorectal cancer. Toward the end, he regretted having had as much chemotherapy as he did; he felt if he had refused part of those treatments, he might have died a little sooner, but he would have had more time where he could enjoy life.

The medical establishment is so geared to an all-out effort to preserve life that it is hard to get them to back off when that is appropriate. The whole hospice movement has developed to deal with this problem and is a good answer for many people with terminal illnesses like cancer where the end is slow and (relatively) predictable.

So far the legislative response to the end of life problem has generally been limited to encouraging hospice and similar programs as an option that people can take and providing for advance medical directives and similar devices where people can express their intentions in advance. Both are useful, but have their limitations. In the end, each person's circumstances are unique. At some point in many cases the all-out medical effort to preserve life becomes high tech torture that does the patient no good. Calling an end at that point is one of the toughest decisions any of us will ever have to make — possibly for ourselves, but more likely for a parent or our spouse.

We had a circumstance in our neighborhood a few years ago that illustrated the problem. One of our neighbors had a terminal cancer. During his third hospitalization, he decided there was no point in going on, summoned his lawyer and his accountant, made sure his affairs were in order, ordered the advance life support turned off and died 48 hours later. One of my neighbors summed it up well, "You know, James did the right thing. He saved himself a lot of suffering and his family a lot of money. But if it was me, I don't know if I'd have had the guts to do it."

In this area I think it is unwise for the government to try to intervene. It is inappropriate for the government to either ration care or do the opposite and force patients to receive care. I think the best we can do is set up the system so patients and their families can make their own decisions. We should keep the government, particularly the courts, from second guessing decisions made in good faith.

All these steps will be, by themselves, only partly effective. What we know demonstrates three causes for unnecessary care: 1) economic with providers making money by keeping otherwise idle resources busy, 2) defensive medicine induced by our tort liability system, and 3) meeting patients' and doctors' expectations that no stone will be left unturned in a circumstance where scientific evidence on what is really needed is either absent or ignored.

My conclusion, which is not yet supported by sufficient evidence, is that curing all three causes will be necessary before most unnecessary care stops.

Chapter 5, Footnotes

(1) C. Northcote Parkinson, <u>Parkinson's Law</u>, The Riverside Press, 1957, page 2.

(2) The Wall Street Journal, December 22, 2003, page 1.

(3) Richard D. Lamm, <u>The Brave New World of Health Care</u>, Fulcrum Publishing, 2003, page 118. Richard Lamm is a former governor of Colorado.

(4) Jennifer Corbett Dooren, "Colonoscopy May Be Overused As Follow-up to Some Surgery," The Wall Street Journal, August 18, 2004, page D2.

(5) Summary of Health Care Problems in Wyoming, by the Select Committee on Health Care, prepared by the Legislative Service Office, August 1991, page 4.

(6) Fisher et. al., Annals of Internal Medicine, 2003, 138, pages 273-287 and 288-298.

(7) Fisher, Ibid, page 273.

(8) Fisher, Ibid, page 288.

(9) Fisher, Ibid, page 288

(10) Sheila Leatherman and Douglas McCarthy, "Quality of Health Care in the United States: A Chartbook," Chart 1-8 Appropriateness of Procedures as Rated by Expert Consensus, page 38. Published by The Commonwealth Fund, April 2002.

(11) David M. Cutler, <u>Your Money or Your Life: Strong Medicine for America's Health Care System</u>, Oxford University Press, 2004, page 58. The sources Cutler cites as his authority are from reputable, peer reviewed journals, principally the New England Journal of Medicine and the Annals of Internal Medicine.

(12) Leatherman and McCarthy, Ibid, page 38.

(13) Kessler D., McCellan, M., "Do Doctors Practice Defensive Medicine," Quarterly Journal of Economics, 111 (2): 353-390, 1996.

(14) Lamm, Ibid, pages 117 & 118.

(15) Alex Frangos, "Model vs. Model, A comparison of countries' healthcare systems," The Wall Street Journal, February 21, 2001, page R4.

(16) Frangos, Ibid, page R4.

(17) Fisher et al., Ibid, page 291.

(18) David F. Crowder, M.D., Crowder Consulting Group, Ltd, presentation entitled "Help me Doctor! I've been billed and I can't get up," given to the Wyoming Legislature's Joint Interim Labor, Health and Social Services Committee, July 23, 2002.

(19) Chapter 225, Session Laws of Wyoming, 1987.

Chapter 6

COST SHIFTING

Cost shifting is a major fact of life in the American health care system and one of the important reasons the cost of health insurance is rising faster than the cost of health care.

Cost shifting can be best understood in the hospital setting although it also occurs in other settings. When the hospital treats a patient, it has certain expenses — it has to pay the nurses and the rest of the staff; it has to pay for the medical supplies the patient uses, the utility fees for lighting and heating and many other costs. Suppose that patient doesn't pay or doesn't pay the full cost of the treatment. The hospital still has to pay its bills. If it is going to stay in business, it has to get the money it needs from somewhere. What it does is raise the rates to the paying customers so they are paying more than the cost of serving just them.

Health care is not the only sector in the economy where cost shifting occurs. Shoplifting is an example of cost shifting in the retail sector. Shoplifters get goods without paying; merchants know it happens so they raise the prices to the rest of us a little to cover the cost. What makes health care different is the scale of the problem. In the rest of the economy when someone doesn't pay, they are refused service. In the shoplifting example, as the volume of shoplifting increases merchants take progressively more aggressive steps to stop it.

In health care there are legal and moral obstacles to providers refusing to see patients who don't pay. Our society has decided that nobody who needs acute medical care will be refused due to inability to pay. Hospital emergency rooms are the providers of last resort. As a matter of federal law (currently the act known as EMTALA, the 1985 Emergency Medical Treatment and Labor Act), a hospital emergency room has to treat all patients that show up and appear to have a medical emergency. And if they need it, they have to be admitted to the rest of the hospital, provided the hospital has the ability to treat their problem. There are sanctions for non-compliance including monetary penalties and termination from Medicare and Medicaid.[1]

This started with the old Hill/Burton act that helped finance most hospital construction in the post-World War II era — a hospital that took Hill/Burton funds had to agree to treat all patients regardless of ability to pay as a condition of accepting those funds. This was not a big deal for the hospitals — most of the community hospitals were behaving this way already for ethical reasons. There are various other traditions that got hospitals into the business of treating non-paying patients. For example, teaching hospitals did it to get a supply of patients their interns and residents could practice on. The net result is that in health care if you can't pay, you can still get a major service, something generally not true in the rest of the economy.

The analysis of the cost shifting problem is compounded by the phenomenon of marginal cost pricing. This practice is best understood by looking at the example of the airline industry. If an airplane is going to fly between two cities, it makes almost no difference in the cost whether a seat is full or empty. If an airline can sell an otherwise empty seat at a severely discounted price, it makes more money than if the seat goes empty. That's true provided it is selling a seat that really otherwise would be empty and not just selling a seat at a cut-rate price that would otherwise sell at a full price.

The result has been a very sophisticated pricing system designed to sell discounted tickets to the leisure traveler who would otherwise not go or would drive while sticking the non-discretionary business traveler with the full-price fare. Some of the same phenomenon occurs in health care, but with important differences.

When we in Wyoming considered participating in the child health program, we were planning to reimburse on the Medicaid rate, which is significantly below the provider's total cost. This did not bother the doctors much — they continued to advocate for the program. Their reasoning seemed to be twofold — in part now they would be paid something for a service that they were already providing for free and they would attract some new business from people previously doing without, and that would fill empty beds or take up idle doctor's office time. Since the reimbursement was high enough to pay the additional expenses of seeing another patient (what the economists call the marginal cost), the doctor was money ahead with the new business.

A problem in health care is that the payers expecting marginal cost pricing have too big a market share. The two big government programs, Medicare and Medicaid, usually pay a discounted price and between them they typically have almost half the business, and for some providers, significantly more than half the business. In addition, big HMOs and big insurers with large market shares want discounts and, where there is competition, will shift their business to get it. And unlike the airline example, a full bed is much more expensive for a hospital than an empty bed. And when a hospital brings in a class of low paying patients it can't serve them just when there aren't enough high paying customers like the airlines do. It has to treat them when they need it and size its facility and staff accordingly. And for legal and ethical reasons, providers can't skimp on services for low paying patients — everybody has to get the standard of care including all the expensive tests. The result is that the net effect of government programs that pay less than full cost and others who negotiate discounts is to increase the cost to everybody else.

Cost shifting not only moves the costs from one payer to another, it also increases the total cost of the health care system. By raising private health insurance costs, it increases the number of uninsured people because employees and their employers can no longer afford health insurance. The uninsured get health care in more costly settings. Porter and Teisberg speaking of the cost shifting due to discounts for large plans and large employers explain it very well: "Such cost shifting ultimately drives up overall costs — even to large groups — by increasing the number of uninsured patients who must be treated in expensive settings (emergency rooms for instance) and hence the amount of free care that must be subsidized."[2]

In addition, there is evidence that being uninsured increases costs because the uninsured are less likely to get preventive care and routine care that can keep small medical problems from becoming big ones.[3] Cost shifting from government programs has exactly the same effect except it drives up the costs for everyone else in the system and not the government directly.

The impact of cost shifting is major. In Wyoming I calculated that the average hospital bill for the private pay/private insurance customer is 30 percent higher than the actual cost of providing the service. Our hospitals are running near the break-even point, so very little of that cost is profit; most is cost shifting. I figure the Medicare program alone raises the private bill by 15 percent. This is a big hidden tax because the Congress would rather promise benefits than pay for them. For Medicaid where the rates are set by the state, the figure is five percent. We aren't much more generous than the feds, we just have a much smaller hospital market share.[4] Private bad debt and charity care rounds out the cost shifting at 10 percent.

I caution readers that these figures are crude and subject to some error, although I am confident on average they are close. I developed them by a quick analysis of aggregate hospital data for Wyoming. I would love to see a more careful analysis resulting in better figures. I suspect there are important differences from one kind of health care provider to another and from one service to another. I also caution against using hospital-generated figures on the size of their uncompensated care or bad debt write-offs. These are almost always based on their published prices and have little to do with their actual costs.

When I'm talking to civic groups about the high cost of private health insurance, I say the deadbeats in the system raise the audience's health insurance cost by 30 percent and the biggest deadbeat is the government of the United States in the Medicare program.

In other states these figures will be different from ours in Wyoming. Medicare in particular is not consistent from one state to the next or even one hospital to the next in how well it pays. The differences are major — in September 2002, the U.S. Senate Rural Health Caucus reported, "According to the latest Medicare figures, Medicare's annual inpatient payments per beneficiary by state of residence range from slightly more than $3,000 in predominantly rural states like Wyoming, Idaho and Iowa to over $7,000 in other states."[5]

We get hit particularly hard in Wyoming, but in the majority of states Medicare reimbursement is well below cost. In some of the states, particularly ones on the East and West coasts, Medicare reimbursement is close to actual cost. There were some provisions in the new Medicare law, the one enacted in 2003 that provided the new prescription drug benefit, that were supposed to reduce this problem, but so far I haven't seen any evidence that it has made a significant difference.

Medicaid reimbursement is set by the states and does vary by state. In particular, when a state has financial difficulties, reducing Medicaid reimbursement is a favorite tactic. The resulting cost shifting raises private bills, but that is a well hidden tax and doesn't make the voters mad the way an explicit tax increase does.

In addition, the ability of private groups to negotiate below cost reimbursement varies considerably with local market conditions. We don't see much of that in Wyoming. Our hospitals are all sole community providers and are geographically isolated; our doctors are in short supply. Our providers will not give the kinds of discounts given elsewhere. There are some discounts and the insurance companies often refuse to pay the full bills on the grounds that charges are above the local norm, but our providers face less pressure for discounts than elsewhere due to their quasi monopoly positions. In a suburban setting with a surplus of doctors and competing hospitals, large private payers have considerable negotiating power.

A word on the politics of Medicaid (and probably Medicare) reimbursements. The current below cost reimbursements are a result of an odd political alliance between liberal and conservative politicians. The conservative politicians tend to favor low reimbursements because that cuts down the costs of government and reduces the need for taxes. Conservatives see anything that does that as good. Conservatives tend not to understand cost shifting — the "tax" it causes is well enough hidden that they don't see it. The liberals favor low reimbursements because they are instinctively hostile to wealthy providers and because cheaper costs for government programs that don't make a profit fit their model of how the world ought to work. To the extent they understand the cost shifting they are causing, that doesn't bother them. Anything that raises private insurance costs without raising the cost of government programs is fine with them — it brings us that much closer to a nationalized government-run health system, which is where they want to go.

My experience in Wyoming is that doctors do better at improving reimbursements than hospitals for political reasons. I strongly suspect that other states are similar. Doctors are individuals who vote, contribute to political campaigns, and are often politically active. Hospitals are large bureaucratic entities that can't vote and don't do the other political things that get doctors their political clout. They employ a lot of people, but those people usually don't identify their financial well-being with the political needs of their employer. The result is that while cost shifting from government programs is a problem for both, it is more of a problem for hospitals than doctors.

A result of this cost shifting system is that the highest charges for hospital care go to those who can least afford to pay them. The hospital raises its published charges to try to recover the cost shifting. The ones that pay the published charges are the insurers without enough market share to successfully demand a discount and the uninsured. A few of the uninsured are wealthy, but most are uninsured because they are poor. As the hospitals get in financial trouble, they get aggressive about collecting from such people.

In 2003 and 2004, The Wall Street Journal has run occasional articles on this problem with stories of the problems this practice is causing for some of our most vulnerable citizens. They often draw on New York state examples. In New York, there is a state program that reimburses hospitals for part of their uncompensated care, but it requires the hospitals to make efforts to collect from those who haven't paid, adding a state bureaucratic mandate to the financial incentives the hospitals already have.[6]

What happens when health care costs increase as they are now? Just because 30 percent of the private hospital bill comes from cost shifting, it is not necessarily true that cost shifting will cause 30 percent of increases in health care costs to be shifted; significantly more may be shifted. It depends on the behavior of the entities doing the cost shifting.

For the private bad debt cases, the behavior is clear. They couldn't pay their bills when the bills were smaller. There is no reason to think they will be able to pay any significant amount of an increase in their bills. In fact in 2001 through 2003 due to the recession, the absolute amount they could pay has probably gone down. Therefore virtually all the increase in costs for this group is being cost shifted.

The picture for the Medicaid program for where the states set the reimbursement level is also grim. In 2003 all but a handful of states had deficits to deal with and for about half of them the deficits were serious. As of 2004, the improving economy is starting to help state finances, but most states still have budget problems. A number of states have cut Medicaid reimbursements. Most of the rest are holding the line. Very few have raised reimbursements. The state of Wyoming is one of the few exceptions. In 2002 and 2003, we raised reimbursements for doctors and nursing homes but not hospitals. The net result is that in most states, the medical inflation cost increases for services provided by Medicaid have been cost shifted.

The case of Medicare is less clear. In the late 1990s the federal government cut many Medicare reimbursements as part of its effort to balance the budget. These cuts generated enough political heat that they have been at least in part reversed. In addition, there are some complicated formulas involved in the calculation of reimbursements. A careful study would be required to calculate the real impact of medical inflation on Medicare cost shifting, and I am unaware of any such study. My guess is that a significant portion of the medical inflation cost increases for services to Medicare patients is being cost shifted.

The net outcome is that private health insurance is bearing not only the medical inflation on the cost of the services it consumes, but a significant portion of the medical inflation on the governmental and bad debt care. Cost shifting is the principal source of the difference between medical inflation and the health care cost increases experienced by large self-insured employers, at least for the low end of the range of those cost increases. It is a major, but not the only factor for the small employers.

Chapter 6, Footnotes

(1) Presentation to NCSL fall meeting, December 12, 2003, by Barbara Marone, Federal Affairs Director, American College of Emergency Physicians.

(2) Michael E. Porter and Elizabeth Olmstead Teisberg, "Redefining Competition in Health Care," Harvard Business Review, June 2004, pages 68 & 69.

(3) See "The Cost of Not Covering the Uninsured, Project Highlights," The Kaiser Commission on Medicaid and the Uninsured, June 2003, and "A Shared Destiny, Community Effects of Uninsurance," Institute of Medicine, 2003.

(4) In total, the Medicaid program is almost the same size as the Medicare program, but Medicaid is the majority of the market in long-term care where Medicare is a minor player. Medicare has a much larger share of the acute care market.

(5) Letter dated September 16, 2002, to Chairman Baucus and ranking member Grassley of the Senate Committee on Finance, signed by Senators Craig Thomas and Tom Harkin, co-chairs, Senate Rural Health Caucus and 42 other members of the Rural Health Caucus.

(6) See Lucette Lagnado, "Dunned for Old Bills, Poor Find Some Hospitals Never Forget," The Wall Street Journal, June 8, 2004, page 1, and Lucette Lagnado, "Hospital Found 'Not Charitable' Loses its Status as Tax Exempt," The Wall Street Journal, February 19, 2004, page B1.

Chapter 7

INSURANCE PROBLEMS

The previous chapter showed cost shifting is an important reason that the cost of health coverage has risen faster than the medical inflation rate. But it doesn't account for all the higher increases, especially for the small group and individual markets. This chapter will discuss a number of other problems that are causing increases in the cost of health care coverage. The problems include adverse selection, cyclical factors, state coverage mandates and other regulatory costs.

Adverse selection is always an important concern in the insurance business. Adverse selection happens when the decisions that people make in buying insurance results in a particular company or a particular line of insurance receiving an undue percentage of the bad risks.

At the risk of being too elementary for a couple of paragraphs, let me explain. We buy insurance to have the financial resources to deal with a risk that may happen to us and will be very expensive if it does. The insurance company charges us a premium that is based on the average risk that the bad thing will happen, plus their administrative costs and profit. The people who are lucky and avoid the bad outcome pay for the people who are unlucky and incur the expense. For a given amount of cost in bad outcomes, the more lucky people the lower the premium.

When all goes well in the market, everybody is better off — the insurance company makes money and we have traded the cost of the bad outcome, which we can't afford for the average risk that we can afford. The problem comes when something goes wrong in the marketplace so that only the people who are bad risks buy the insurance. Then there aren't enough lucky people to pay for the unlucky ones and premiums go up. That's adverse selection.

Insurance companies go to great lengths to identify and prevent adverse selection. If they can identify bad risks, they can either charge them more or avoid them. A rate difference based on tobacco use for either life or health insurance is an example of charging a bad risk more. Using tobacco significantly increases your risk of expensive health problems and early death. Insurance companies often charge tobacco users higher premiums. As a marketing strategy they may express it as a discount for being tobacco-free, but the effect is the same — you pay more if you use tobacco.

If insurance companies don't realize they are getting too many bad risks, then they can lose money or even be forced out of business. If they knowingly get stuck with too many bad risks that their competitors avoid, then they have to raise their premiums and become uncompetitive in the marketplace. This is why auto insurance companies want to know about your driving record. Having accidents or moving violations means that you are at higher risk for another accident.

The insurance company wants to know that so they can charge you a higher premium. Charging the bad risks a higher premium means that they can charge the good risks a lower premium. An insurance company that doesn't act this way when its competitors are will promptly be victimized by adverse selection. It will be charging the bad risks a lower rate for their business and it will get their business. It will be charging the good risks a higher rate than the competitors and will lose their business.

A different problem arises when insurance companies are kept from identifying bad risks. If we can prevent the insurance companies from learning what people's driving records are, then they will have to charge the good drivers and the bad drivers the same premium. The rates for the bad drivers will come down and the rates for the good drivers will go up. We sometimes see legislation of this nature — forbidding the release of information on people's moving violations to insurance companies is a typical example. Such bills are usually brought by legislators with a lead foot and the speeding tickets to prove it or who have influential constituents with the same problem. The rest of us usually vote such bills down — unless the bad risk involved is one most people have or one that people can't avoid with better behavior.

Health insurance is like any other insurance — the risks are not evenly distributed. A good rule of thumb is that 20 percent of the insureds will cause 80 percent of the expense.

Halvorson and Isham in their excellent book, Epidemic of Care, report that one percent of the insureds will cause 30 percent of the expense.[1] The ability to predict the bad health risks, particularly on a yearly basis, is good and getting better. An insurance company that can avoid the bad risks can charge the good risks less and make more money than one that can't.

In a totally unregulated small group and individual marketplace, the ability to identify bad risks and not insure them will overwhelm all other factors as a determinant of health insurance company profitability. The marketplace would rapidly bankrupt any insurance company that did not use this ability skillfully and thoroughly. The result in such an unregulated insurance market would be that the bad risks would lose their health insurance either because they were denied coverage or because they could not afford it. As a society, we have decided everyone will get acute care so if the rest of us don't pay for the bad risks in higher insurance premiums, we will pay for them in higher health costs due to cost shifting.

Also, as discussed in the previous chapter, being uninsured increases health care costs, so we will pay more. And there is the social cost of driving people to bankruptcy due to their health care bills. And all of us have some chance of becoming a bad risk. So for health insurance we are willing to legislate to keep insurance companies from responding to the marketplace and discriminating too much against the bad risks.

For large employers adverse selection is usually not a major problem. It is true that people who have a health risk will seek employers who offer insurance while this benefit is not as important to some who don't think they have a risk. This gives some risk of adverse selection, but employers hire on the basis of ability to do the job they need done. They get their share of the bad risks, but not more than their share. For a combination of legal, ethical, and labor relations reasons they cannot deny the bad risks insurance while offering it to the good risks. Their decision to offer or not offer health insurance is based on competitive factors in the labor market, collective bargaining agreements and social conscience. The net effect is relatively little adverse selection for large employer health insurance.

It is possible for a large employer to induce adverse selection. If they charge the employee too much premium for coverage or, more likely, too much premium for dependent coverage, they can induce the healthy risks to leave their insurance plan, raising the per member costs for everyone else.

Our Wyoming State employees' health insurance plan had this kind of adverse selection for dependent coverage. We "solved" the problem with money — we decided to pay 85 percent of the cost of dependent insurance and cut our share of what we pay for the employees from 100 percent to 85 percent. With the employees paying only 15 percent of the cost of the coverage, it's unlikely we will save enough on the employees and insure enough more low risk dependents to lower the state's total cost. Certainly we had to appropriate more money.

I think we have lowered the per-person cost of the insurance, but increased the total cost by insuring more dependents. By offering a better benefit package, we have improved our competitiveness in the employee marketplace for all but the single people with no dependents. Whether we improved it enough to justify the extra cost is something reasonable people can and will disagree about.

For small employers, adverse selection is a much more important factor. What's different for small employers is the motivation for the decision to purchase health insurance. If the owner or a key employee or one of their dependents has a health risk, the employer will provide health insurance. If they are all young and healthy, she may decide health insurance costs too much, and use the money saved to pay higher salaries or grow the business. Since only 58 percent of employers with 3-9 employees and 76 percent of those with 10-24 employees offer health insurance nationally,[2] there is clearly a major opportunity for adverse selection.

By 1990 the insurance companies were dealing with adverse selection in the small group market by refusing to insure companies with bad risks or having the same effect by raising their prices through the ceiling. The social costs of depriving people of health insurance due to this practice were too high, so the states responded with laws requiring guarantee issue (the insurers have to insure all who apply) in the small group market and putting restrictions on pricing.

The federal Congress in 1996 followed the state lead with a law (part of the HIPPA act) requiring guarantee issue nationally in the small group market.

The guarantee issue provision enshrines in law the opportunity for adverse selection. No matter how bad the health risks, the small employer can get insurance. I think the costs of allowing the bad risks to go uninsured justify the guarantee issue law, and I'm one of those who caused it to happen. In Wyoming in 1992, my committee sponsored and I pushed through the relevant law and we were the second state in the nation to do so.[3]

The pricing restrictions are a key part of the guaranteed issue law. It's clear that if the prices are unrestrained, the guaranteed issue requirement is meaningless — the insurance companies can price the bad risk employee groups out of the market. The feds have left this issue to the states and the states' approaches have differed. Colorado tried a community rating approach. In community rating, everyone pays the same price although some variation may be allowed for factors like age. What happened in Colorado was adverse selection on a grand scale. The healthy risks left the small group market and either went uninsured or bought their insurance in the individual market. Small group premiums exploded because so many of the remaining insureds had major risks.[4]

A more common solution has been rate bands. With a band, the rate charged an employer may not vary from an index rate by more than a set percentage. Legislating the percentage is tricky. Set it too low and like Colorado you will induce adverse selection as the healthy risks leave. Set it too high and some of the businesses with high risks can no longer afford the insurance. In Wyoming we had set the percentage at 25 percent and in 2003 we raised it to 35 percent to reduce the adverse selection. The information we had was that the 25 percent rate was the most common among states with a rate band, but 35 percent was used by some. I sponsored the change because our small group insurance rates were growing so fast I thought we almost certainly had a major adverse selection problem, but I will be the first to admit it's hard to prove whether we did the right thing or not.

Except for Colorado's special circumstance, I have never seen reliable numbers on how important the adverse selection problem is in the small group market. I have spoken to a number of the academic experts in the area and they have either said they don't have the data or denied the problem exists. I think adverse selection was not a major problem in the mid-'90s when health care cost increases were mild, but has become one in more recent years as the cost increases have taken off again. Because of the time lags in data collection and academic analysis, the academic experts don't yet have a fix on the problem. My sense is that at least for the small group market, its impact is major.

For the individual insurance market, adverse selection is potentially an overwhelming problem. For the small group market, there is some mixture of good and bad risks in each group, mitigating the impact of the bad risks in most cases. The individual market doesn't even have this mitigation. The result is that most states have not tried guaranteed issue for the individual market. We allow insurance companies to refuse bad risks, at least for the initial sale.

Renewals are treated differently, but they don't carry the degree of adverse selection risk new sales do. This approach leaves bad risks uninsured with all the problems that causes, but most of us fear that the guarantee issue alternative would cause individual insurance to be unavailable for everybody, not just the bad risks. This happened in Washington state in the early 1990s. Many states (including Wyoming) have a subsidized high-risk pool for those who can't get individual insurance, but these often cost so much they are of limited value.

The insurance cycle is another factor blamed for causing health insurance prices to rise faster than health care costs. The basic argument is that there is less competition than there used to be in the health insurance market so there is less competitive restraint on the ability of insurance companies to raise prices. This is clearly true to some degree, and is especially true in some states where unwise regulation or regulation designed to protect a local monopoly provider has driven out too many of the competitors.

In addition the 9/11 attack and a number of natural disasters are having an effect on the insurance market. The amount of insurance a company can write is limited by the amount of capital it has. Regulators and market based self policing through ratings from companies like A.M. Best enforce limits to make sure the companies will have enough resources to meet their obligations. The disasters cost the insurance industry generally a significant portion of its capital. Less capital means less insurance can be written, reducing competition. Companies have therefore been able to raise prices. The effect in health insurance has been largely secondary — reinsurance rates have risen and some companies have redeployed assets from health insurance to other more profitable lines.

Interest rates are another cyclical factor that has affected insurance markets. There is a time lag between when premiums are taken in and benefits are paid out. During this time lag, the premiums are invested. Capital and reserves also are invested. The income from the investments reduces the size of the premiums that must be charged. In the past few years interest rates and investment returns in general have gone way down as anyone with a 401(k) or an IRA knows all too well. Insurance companies have been hit just like most other investors. This has been less of a problem for health insurance companies than others because the time lag between when the premium comes in and the benefits are paid is less than for some other kinds of insurance, but it is still a contributor to rising health insurance costs.

All three of these cyclical factors have converged to give us a "hard" market for all lines of insurance. In a hard market, insurance companies can and do raise rates more than their underlying costs would seem to justify. I have not found a reliable analysis of how much of a contributor to higher rates these cyclical factors are, but my sense is they are third in importance to cost shifting and adverse selection.

Mandates often are accused of being a major source of health insurance increases. State legislatures have developed the bad habit of mandating that health insurance cover a number of items that it otherwise would not. These extras increase the cost of health insurance. They do not affect the cost of coverage that is provided by employers who are self-insured — the states are forbidden to regulate such coverage by the federal Employee Retirement Income Security Act (ERISA). They are one of the reasons that insurance provided through insurance companies is more expensive than ERISA coverage and that insurance costs are going up faster than medical inflation.

The form of mandates varies considerably depending on the specific mandate and the state. Sometimes the mandate just requires that an item be covered like other health aspects of health care. A mental health parity mandate is typically of this nature. It requires that treatment for mental illness be covered to the same extent that treatment for other illness is. Other times the mandate will require that the insurance company pay the full cost without regard to deductibles or co-payments required for other services. A mandate for cancer screening is likely to be of this nature.

Opponents of mandates point to states like Maryland where the process has gotten out of hand. PricewaterhouseCoopers, citing a federal General Accounting Office (GAO), report states that in Maryland mandates add 22 percent to the cost of health insurance.[5] I'm skeptical about the size of this claim — in Wyoming we have very few mandates and high health insurance costs — but I'm in no position to argue with the GAO.

Mental health parity is a commonly proposed and controversial mandate. The argument for it is simple — why should mental health be singled out and covered to a lesser degree than other illnesses? Conventional insurance policies often do just that and it amounts to discrimination against people with mental illness.

Originally there was a good case for the insurance companies limiting their coverage of mental illness. There were two problems. First, the diagnosis of mental illness was not that clear-cut. There were some individuals who very clearly had a mental illness, but there was a big gray area where it was difficult to say if a person was really mentally ill. Second, the treatments for mental illness were not that effective. There weren't many drugs that did any good; the few surgical options available were quite controversial, and psychotherapy was very expensive, didn't always work and lacked clearly defined parameters to judge what was needed.

Insurance companies were faced with a large cost that was hard to control and might not do the customer much good. Limiting the coverage for mental illness was the sensible solution to the problem. That kept health insurance affordable without much harm done to insureds.

The world has changed and is rapidly changing even more. There is a revolution in our ability to diagnose and treat mental illness. Our understanding of the physical, often biochemical, basis of mental illness is growing rapidly. The revolution is not yet complete and there is still a diagnosis problem on the margin, but the old justification of limiting mental health coverage is disappearing. There is a growing array of drugs which, while often very expensive, do work. The need for psychotherapy has not disappeared with the advent of the drugs. For many mental illnesses, a combination of drugs and therapy works best. My theory is that once the drugs have controlled the underlying illness, then the individual is left with an accumulation of mental problems that were originally caused by the illness. Once the illness is controlled, these can be dealt with by therapy. In addition, therapy is getting better at treating mental problems caused by abuse, including sexual abuse, traumatic events in people's lives and substance abuse. There is still a problem of how much is enough with therapy, and the recommendations of experts and professional organizations on that question cannot be free of conflict of interest concerns.

The best figures I can find are that a mental health parity mandate will add between one-half of one percent and one percent to the cost of health insurance. At a time of exploding health insurance costs, adding this much cost will deprive some people of all health coverage and cause others to pay more in deductibles or co-payments that are personally difficult for them. It is important to understand that most health insurance has some coverage for mental illness; it is just more limited than the coverage for physical illnesses. The mental health advocates will disagree, but there is still a reasonable dispute as to whether a mental health parity mandate should be enacted. However, the time is coming when such a mandate will be clearly justified.

The motivation for some mandates can be the economic interest of some politically effective group of providers or patients who want a particular service. I would put a mandate for chiropractic services or special infertility treatments in this category.

Some mandates can be quite expensive. For example mandated chemical dependency treatment coverage has been reported to have increased costs by nine percent.[6] Pricewaterhouse claims that a mandate for routine dental services increased costs by 15 percent.[7] This kind of a mandate is a mistake. Routine dental care is something that most people who can get insurance can afford on their own. It involves a lot of small claims and on those the insurance company administrative costs are likely to be high. People can reasonably decide it will be cheaper to pay for their routine dental costs directly, so the state ought to stay out of that decision.

Other mandates make more sense. Take breast cancer screening. Early detection of breast cancer unquestionably saves lives. There is controversy and individual variation over which treatment is best once cancer is detected, but all the standard treatments are effective and are more effective the earlier the cancer is detected. There is some controversy about the age at which mass screening is justified and the individual circumstances justifying screening at an earlier age, but for most women there are clear guidelines.

A mandate for breast cancer screening adds some costs to insurance coverage, both for the screening and for the prompt treatment when the screening finds cancer. For those cases detected early, it saves the money that would eventually be spent on the often futile but very expensive treatment of advanced breast cancer. Given the extent people have to change insurance coverages, the savings in individual cases may accrue to a different company than the one that incurs the screening expense, but all ought to benefit from the general savings to the system, unless the real savings beneficiary is Medicare.

There is good argument that there is a more effective way than a health insurance mandate for increasing the amount of breast cancer screening. The insurance mandate does not reach those covered by ERISA-exempt coverage, the uninsured and those on Medicare or Medicaid. Given our screwed up payment system, it may cause excessive insurance administrative costs. I suspect a careful analysis would show that providing breast cancer screening as a free public health service would be more efficient and effective than doing it through an insurance mandate. However, the tax by doing it as an insurance mandate is hidden and the insurance companies take the blame. Free public health benefits are paid for with general taxes for which legislators take the blame. It should be no surprise many legislators prefer the mandate approach.

A further problem in analyzing the cost of a breast cancer screening mandate is that people want it and the marketplace demands this service be part of health insurance coverage. Should all the costs of breast cancer screening paid for by insurance companies be ascribed to this mandate or only the costs for the additional screening caused by the mandate? And what are those additional costs? Are there any or would all the costs be incurred anyway due to marketplace demand?

A further problem with the mandate is caused by political correctness. Breast cancer is 99 percent-plus a female problem; nobody wants to give males mammograms; the male cases are much too rare. Prostate cancer is the male problem. Legislators naturally think that if we mandate breast cancer screening to help the women, to be fair we ought to mandate prostate cancer screening to help the men. The Wyoming Legislature thought this way and we passed both mandates together in the same bill.[8]

The reaction sounds logical and fair. The problem is that unlike breast cancer screening, there is major uncertainty about the value of prostate cancer screening. The test, the Prostate Specific Antigen (PSA), is controversial, accused of too high a rate of both false positives and false negatives.[9] There is controversy over what level of result should trigger additional testing. The PSA itself is risk-free and relatively cheap, but the next stage, an invasive biopsy, is more expensive and any invasive procedure has some risk. And there is major controversy over what to do if prostate cancer is found.

Prostate cancer is a major killer of men, but it is also very common, especially in older men, and frequently causes no trouble. Many men will die of something else long before their prostate cancer causes any problems. The standard interventions have serious side effects and risks. If medical science could easily separate the prostate cancers that are likely to spread and cause trouble from those that are not, screening would make more sense, but this is an advance medical science has not made yet.

The prostate screening mandate therefore makes a lot less sense than the breast cancer one, but in the current political climate it is difficult for a legislature to do one without the other.

There are some other factors that increase the cost of health insurance more than the underlying health care costs are rising. For the most part, they are relatively minor, but they deserve a quick mention.

State insurance departments regulate health insurance and regulation costs money. All states regulate financial solvency to ensure that the insurance company will have the financial resources to pay the claims. If this wasn't done, sooner or later customers would be hurt either by a company that had honestly underestimated its costs and lacked the resources to pay the claims or by outright frauds. Because of the time lag between the payment and the benefit, insurance is unusually vulnerable to fraud. In what other business can a company take your money now and not provide you anything tangible in return until some uncertain time in the future?

Also the states have guarantee funds to assess the solvent companies to pay off the claims of an insolvent one. These two protections are lacking in areas where the federal government has pre-empted state regulation. People who are getting their health coverage from such an unregulated source needs to pay attention to the financial solvency of whoever is providing the insurance — you do not have the protections (or the costs) of state regulation.

All states also deal with customer complaints against insurance companies. This is a major activity for state insurance departments. Insurance policies are contracts, so theoretically you could settle an argument with an insurance company by taking them to court, but normally the legal system is so expensive this is not a practical solution. Instead you call your state insurance department and they will look at your problem and, if the facts justify it, force the company to pay what it owes.

This is another major benefit to having state-regulated insurance — if you have a row with a third party administrator for a self-insured employer or with some other form of health care coverage that the feds have exempted from state regulation, you are on your own. The state insurance department may be sympathetic, but it doesn't have the legal authority to do anything. This protection does add a little to health insurance premiums for state-regulated insurance.

States often also tax insurance premiums. One simple thing state legislatures could do to reduce the cost of health insurance would be to repeal the premium tax. A state that is funding its uninsurable pool by allowing the assessments to support the pool to be deducted from the premium tax as Wyoming is, would have to find a different source of revenue for that purpose. That would be a good idea as using an assessment on insurance companies to support the uninsurable pool is unfair because ERISA-exempt coverage escapes the assessment. These assessments contribute to the higher insurance costs of small businesses and individuals.

States also may assess the insurance companies to provide the funds to run the state insurance departments and these costs are passed to the customers.

Many states regulate the premium rates charged for health insurance premiums. This adds costs both for the insurance companies that have to prepare complicated rate filing documents and for the insurance departments that have to review them. We in Wyoming have avoided this — we figure the marketplace will do a much more efficient job of regulating insurance premiums.

In May 2003 I attended a meeting put on jointly by the Reforming States Group (RSG, a voluntary group of legislators and state administrators interested in health care issues) and the National Association of Insurance Commissioners (NAIC). One of the things we were looking for at that meeting was a regulatory scheme that was getting customers consistently better premium prices. We didn't find one.

All these factors do add to the cost of health insurance, especially compared to the costs incurred by self-insured entities. Except for premium taxes and possibly in some states high-risk pool assessments, they are relatively minor and provide consumer protections worth the cost. Except for the high-risk pool assessments and taxes that are a percentage of the premium, there is no reason any of these should be going up faster than general inflation.

Chapter 7, Footnotes

(1) George C. Halvorson and George J. Isham, Epidemic of Care, Jossey-Bass, 2003, page 41.

(2) "Trends and Indicators in the Changing Health Care Marketplace, 2002, Chartbook," May 2002, The Henry J. Kaiser Family Foundation, page 18. The percentages are for 2001.

(3) Chapter 58, Session Laws of Wyoming, 1992.

(4) Presentation of Colorado Insurance Commissioner to National Conference of State Legislatures, Annual Meeting, Denver Colorado, 2002.

(5) PriceWaterhouseCoopers, "The Factors Fueling Rising Health Care Costs," prepared for the American Association of Health Plans, April 2002, pages 6-7. The study cited is the GAO, "Health Insurance Regulation: Varying State Requirements Affect Cost of Insurance," August 1996.

(6) Ibid, page 6. The study cited is Gail A. Jensen and Michael Morrisey, "Employer-Sponsored Health Insurance and Mandated Benefit Laws," The Milbank Quarterly, Vol. 77, No. 4, 1999.

(7) PriceWaterhouseCoopers, Ibid, page 7.

(8) Chapter 28, Session Laws of Wyoming, 1998.

(9) See Laura Johannes, "Tiny Protein May Lead to Better Test for Prostate Cancer," The Wall Street Journal, November 4, 2003, p. B1. The article cites the National Cancer Institute as the authority for saying that 15 out of 100 men over age 50 will have elevated PSA levels, but 12 of these will not have cancer and three will, while 25-30 percent of PSA tests will be false negatives.

Chapter 8

COMPETITION IN HEALTH CARE

One of the themes in many health care reform proposals is a recommendation to increase or improve competition. Such recommendations often come from economists and others who believe in free markets as the solution to all economic ills. The health care system isn't working very well now. It must therefore have barriers (probably governmental) to free competition. If the marketplace can be restructured so providers and insurance companies can compete freely, all will be well. The assumption is competition will focus the marketplace on enhancing value, which is defined as a combination of price and quality.

Porter and Teisberg in a Harvard Business Review article entitled, "Redefining Competition in Health Care," provide a recent example. The editor summarized the article, "The wrong kinds of competition have made a mess of the American health care system. The right kinds of competition can straighten it out."[1]

Another common idea is that providers or insurance companies are getting monopoly prices so we can reduce prices by getting rid of these monopolies. There is a whole body of antitrust law as applied to health care that is dedicated to this proposition.

The dedication to competition is understandable. It works well in most of our society. To quote Porter and Teisberg, "In healthy competition, relentless improvements in processes and methods drive down costs. Product and service quality rise steadily. Innovation leads to new and better approaches, which diffuse widely and rapidly. Uncompetitive providers are restructured or go out of business. Value-adjusted prices fall, and the market expands."[2]

The personal computer market is an example of market competition at its best of which most of us are familiar, but it is only one example among many. Based on their experiences with the rest of the economy, experts think competition in health care can produce the same results.

We are seeing some of the benefits the experts expect from competition. Our ability to perform medical miracles is expanding rapidly. We can now diagnose and cure many conditions that sent our ancestors to their graves. Our ability to do things like replacing knees and hips has allowed many people to lead much more enjoyable lives. Modern imaging technology has diffused rapidly through our communities allowing doctors to diagnose many conditions with precision. Hospitals that failed to keep up with the high tech advances have been restructured or have gone out of business.

However, when it comes to value and price, watch out for competition in health care. There are circumstances where competition will drive prices down and quality up as it does in the rest of the economy, but there are more circumstances where it will have the opposite effect and drive prices up and hurt quality. The forces driving health care markets are different from those in the rest of the economy. Understanding those differences is very important.

There is a story of a group of doctors in California in the fee-for-service days, which illustrates an important difference. It seems the doctors were making plenty of money, but they were working harder than they wanted to. They didn't have time to enjoy the fruits of their labors. One of the partners, who had taken a freshman economics course in college, suggested, "We ought to raise our prices. Higher prices will reduce the volume of business, so we won't have as many patients. We can have the extra time off we want and our incomes won't come down very much."

The others thought this was a good plan so they did it. The problem was that their volume of business went up so they made even more money, but they had even less time off for their families and hobbies.

This story may be apocryphal, but it rings true and illustrates an important point. In most of the economy when the price of something goes up, people will increasingly say it's not worth the extra cost and will stop buying it or buy less of it. This is the engine that drives business to try to lower the price at the same time they are increasing quality. It is true of everything from beef steak to washing machines. It is even true of highly addictive substances like tobacco. It is especially true in some of the high tech fields like computers, and health care is increasingly high tech with a high rate of technical innovation, but we don't see the same results in improving prices in health care.

Health care is different. We know that the quality of our life, maybe even the continuation of our life, can depend on the quality of the health care we get, and we rightly put a high value on that. We are conditioned by our experiences with the rest of our economy to equate high prices with quality. We know that isn't always true, but it often is. When it comes to health care, we often prefer the more expensive service on the theory it is better and we are willing to pay the higher price to get better. This is especially true when we are spending the money of some third-party payer, like an insurance company or the government, but it is even true with our own money. By raising their prices, the California doctors were sending a signal that they were better quality and that attracted more patients.

The same phenomenon makes it hard to get the patient to control the use of extra medical services. The doctor tells a patient we need another series of tests or an MRI, "just to be on the safe side," and the patient is likely to agree. The reasoning is that if it's my life, being on the safe side is a very good idea. This tendency will be more pronounced when someone else is paying, but will be present even if the patient is paying himself.

In the rest of the economy, higher quality does bring higher prices. Traditionally a Rolls Royce is worth more than a Cadillac, which is in turn worth more than a Chevy because the quality is better. A lot of effort goes into evaluating the quality, and the consumer is in a good position to judge if the extra quality justifies the higher price. And, very importantly, it is very clear how and from whom to get the higher quality.

This is not true in health care. Of course, the patient can tell if he gets better or worse. However in many cases, the patient would get better no matter what the health care system did. In others, the patient will die even if given the best possible care. And in chronic diseases, the quality of care makes a difference over so many years the individual consumer is often in no position to judge from his outcome rapidly enough to do any good in selecting a provider.

Quality can in theory be judged from data about the outcomes various providers produce. However, there are some practical problems, some of which can be solved and some of which cannot. The underlying health status of patients obviously makes a big difference in the outcomes achieved. The very best doctors and hospitals often have worse results because they get the toughest cases. Risk adjustment must be used to compensate for this, and it is difficult to do well and often is subject to controversy.

The variety of human diseases is so wide that frequently, outside of a few common problems, an individual provider or organization will have too few cases to judge their outcomes in a statistically valid way. And there is the time problem with chronic diseases — an improvement made this year may not show up in the outcomes data for five, 10 or even 20 years. The way to get around this is to use process measures. For example, did diabetics have a regular A1c test? But it isn't really the same as outcomes. In the diabetes case, measuring the rate of A1c testing tells you nothing about how effectively problems that the test identified were managed.

And there are also structural barriers to obtaining good data. Providers are reluctant to provide them because of a very real fear such data could be used against them in malpractice lawsuits. And they know such data could hurt them economically or force changes that could be personally uncomfortable.

One question we have to ask about competition in health care is what kind of competition we will get. In the general economy there are several ways firms can compete. They can compete on price, on service, on quality of product, on dozens of factors. Typically, competition is a mixture of these factors with different segments of the market preferring different mixtures. Some people want the prestige and quality of a Cadillac, some want the economy of a Hyundai, and some prefer the prefer the mid-range compromise that is the Chevy.

For all of these choices, the fact of price competition puts an upper limit on what can be offered and the customer's sense of minimum quality (along with government regulations) puts a limit on how cheap the product can be. And for all these choices there is relentless market pressure that has improved the value of the product. In health care, however, price can drop out of the equation as far as the patient is concerned both due to the third-party payment system and because he perceives more expensive as better in a circumstance where better is what counts.

If two hospitals are competing in a community where the patients or the doctors decide which one gets the business, the hospitals will not compete on the basis of price. They will compete by seeking to attract the best (most expensive) doctors and the most doctors. They will compete for both doctors and patients by having the latest and most expensive technology. A virtual arms race for the newest and best can easily ensue. Unless either third-party payers or government regulations interfere, the price increases involved will not matter much and competition will drive up prices. If the expansions result in extra capacity, the hospitals will raise prices to cover their costs and put pressure on doctors to bring in extra business to keep the facility going. Especially where there is a surplus of physicians, the pressure is likely to be successful and the patients (or more correctly their insurers) will pay for a lot of extra tests and minor procedures.

One of the ways the HMOs were successful in the 1990s was to bring price competition back into this equation. In a community with surplus capacity, they would own or contract for what they needed medically to provide the service. They would use the excess capacity to bid one provider against another and force the price down. They could and did cut out providers who would not be competitive on price. They also tried to rein in the excess utilization. The result was that in the mid-'90s, we had some years where prices in health care were almost flat. However, the providers hated it and the customers (patients) objected to the lack of choice. In separating what was medically necessary from what wasn't, the HMOs made some mistakes that the providers skillfully hyped in the media. The HMOs got cast as villains in the public eye and got restrained by a combination of marketplace and regulatory factors leading to our renewed explosion in prices.

Halvorson and Isham, who are deeply involved in managed care (Halvorson is CEO of Kaiser Permanente, a major national HMO, and Isham is medical director for HealthPartners, a Minnesota HMO), give an excellent account of what went wrong in their book <u>Epidemic of Care</u>. In their chapter on "Care Monopolies," they explain just how local health care markets are and how easy it is for providers to consolidate and provide a united front to beat back HMOs seeking to use price competition to drive down provider reimbursements. The problem for the HMO is that it needs a presence in every geographic part of the market it has entered. By consolidating in a community, those providers can say "if you want to offer services in our community, you have to meet our reimbursement terms."

The market is very geographically fragmented and it has proved relatively easy for the providers to consolidate enough so they, not the HMO, are dictating terms. In their chapter on "Medical Necessity Calls, Fee Cuts, and PR Errors," they describe how some of the HMO attempts to restrain excessive utilization where bungled, exploited by providers mad about fee cuts, and resulted in government regulations and marketplace troubles. With their practical experience, they do a better job than I can in explaining the ins and outs of all this. I commend their book to the reader interested in the specifics.[3]

In Wyoming, competition among hospitals has taken a little different flavor although many of the principles we see in other states apply here as well. Our hospitals are all sole community providers. Except for a few free-standing surgical clinics, they do not have local competition. They still will do many of the same things their urban counterparts do in an effort to compete for doctors. They buy as much of the newest and best equipment as they can. They are competing to keep patients at home who otherwise would have to be referred to a larger hospital outside their community. There are economic, and patient convenience and safety reasons for this.

Some of the economic factors are direct and obvious. Providing a more complete spectrum of medical services locally will mean more jobs in the local economy. Indirectly, offering better and more complete medical services makes the community a more attractive place for new businesses to locate.

Hospital boards are controlled by local business people. They understand these effects and usually have a personal financial interest in the performance of the local economy.

Patient convenience is obvious — who wants to drive a hundred miles to a different community for health care if it could be obtained locally?

Patient safety is less clear, but still a factor. For many conditions, the time to transport a patient to needed care is not a big safety issue, but it is for some emergency conditions. This factor is more important for Wyoming than most other places; we have a population of a half-million scattered over an area larger than New England. Also, in many cases patients will do better in their local community. They will feel more at home and will be more likely to intervene in their own care to prevent errors. They will have better support from family and friends. There is a psychological aspect to medicine, and support can be very important.

Nolen devotes an entire chapter to the advantages of being treated in a community hospital close to home. He says, "It's impossible to overestimate the value to a patient of being in familiar surroundings at times of stress. I've had patients who, I'm sure, survived serious illnesses because they had the support of their friends, their relatives and their clergyman when they were fighting for their lives. Without that sort of support, they'd have given up; and every doctor knows that when a patient gives up, the battle is usually lost."[4]

In sparsely populated areas like Wyoming, there are some effective restraints on how much institutions can expand. One is the effect of volume on patient safety. For many procedures, a certain volume of patients is essential to give the providers enough practice so they can become and remain proficient. The surgeon and OR team who do an "occasional" open heart case are deadly and everyone knows it. The same applies to many other procedures, and the medical staff and hospital administrators are well aware of the basics even though they may sometimes take chances providing services locally that don't quite have enough volume for the local team to have full proficiency

Another factor is the effect of volume on the economics. A specialist needs a certain number of patients to be economically viable. A facility needs a certain volume to cover fixed costs. The government is ineffective at regulating the utilization it pays for and the insurance companies have difficulty keeping prices down, but they do enough to set some practical limits on what can be profitably done. A specialist who lacks enough volume can't raise prices enough to make up the difference.

In the Wyoming setting, I am sure that the desire to provide as much medical service locally as possible leads us to have more facilities than a strictly economically rational system would give us. Given the medical and local economy advantages of local services, I will not say the result is wrong, but it does run our cost up.

Competition among health insurance companies is another factor that can sometimes run prices up. This doesn't sound right on the face of it — one would think that multiple companies competing would drive the price down and the more that were competing, the more the price could be driven down. People, and employers, may not be price sensitive in buying health care, but they sure are when buying health insurance. There are, however, a couple of minor and a couple of major factors that can drive prices up.

The minor ones first. One is that each insurance company has a separate regulatory cost of doing business in each state. It has to be admitted, file reports, get policy forms approved, and, if the state is one that regulates prices, get premium prices approved. These costs are by company and more companies mean more costs. Unless the state insurance department is very difficult to deal with, these costs should be minor.

Another important cost that will go up at least a little with competition is the selling cost. More companies will mean more difficulty marketing. There may need to be more advertising and promotion, and more time will be spent by agents. These costs are real, will be incurred by all companies and have to be covered somehow.

A major cost can be the insurance company's ability to negotiate discounts with providers. Discounts are common in health care and market share counts when negotiating discounts. With too many companies in a market, none of them will have enough market share to get much of a discount from providers. A few companies with big market shares may well be able to get significant discounts. This is particularly true if there is a surplus of providers and there aren't any legal or other obstacles to the insurer for switching patients to the providers with the discounts.

Competition among health insurance companies also can be trouble for people with health problems. Recall the previous discussion that 20 percent of the population incurs 80 percent of the cost and one percent incurs 30 percent of the cost. Health insurers can compete on their ability to avoid the high cost people. Avoiding even a small part of the high cost population will do more for the insurer's profitability than anything it can do to build volume by holding the general costs down. This is the insurance company side of the adverse selection process discussed in the previous chapter.

The government has done two major things to combat this problem. First, as discussed in the previous chapter, there is a guarantee issue provision in the small group market. Second, there is a regulation in the tax code that all employees within a given class must be treated alike for the cost of health insurance to be tax-deductible. Some companies also have discovered that by devices like employee premium shares, they can cause their low wage employees to refuse the insurance. Surprisingly, some employers have discovered the opposite strategy works better. In Wyoming, Natrona County School District #1 has discovered that providing health insurance benefits to part-time, low wage employees like cafeteria workers is a cost effective way to get loyal, long-term employees in those jobs.

The demand for discounts is a particularly troubling issue in health care. We discussed in the previous chapter how a demand for discounts could induce cost shifting that increased costs for everyone. That isn't the whole story, however. A demand for a discount is a demand for price competition and that puts providers under pressure to be more efficient. This is the kind of thing that in the rest of the economy leads to improvements in efficiency and value and forces suppliers unable to match others' efficiencies out of business. I think it was an important element in the rise of managed care and the reduction in the rate of health care cost increases in the 1990s.

Some of the HMOs, particularly the staff model ones, got rid of the excesses of physicians and facilities that lead to unnecessary care. The patient got a cheaper product that did him as much or more good. They were enhancing value, which is exactly what you should expect competition to do. Unfortunately due to the difficulty the customer has in judging value (for example, separating the needed medical services from the unneeded ones) and the cost structure of health care where so few patients are so much of the cost, too many HMOs found that they could compete for business by rationing needed care and by skillful strategies to avoid the sickest patients. The results did not enhance value and got all the HMOs in marketplace and regulatory trouble. I think it may be that given enough time, possibly more time than society has, the HMOs that really enhance value may eventually win out in the competitive marketplace. But so far it hasn't happened on a wide enough scale.

A further problem with insurers using demands for discounts to get price competition is sometimes the government places legal obstacles in the way of the process. Some states use an any willing provider law. We have one in Wyoming.[5] It states that if an insurer negotiates a reduced rate with providers, it must accept into its plan any provider willing to accept that rate. This destroys the insurer's negotiating position — a provider can refuse to participate in negotiating a reduced rate knowing that later he can always accept the rate and opt in.

The insurer can't promise to deliver all his business to those who do negotiate, and he loses his leverage. In the Wyoming case, I believe our law does little harm because our provider community is so thin that there is little incentive to negotiate discounts in return for volume. Most of our doctors already have more volume than they want. In a state with surpluses of providers, such a law could greatly restrict price competition among providers.

There is also a problem that enhancing value for certain kinds of patients is a strategy that gets a provider in financial trouble. Take diabetics. If a capitated provider, like an HMO, does a better job of taking care of diabetics, it runs the risk that the word will get out in the diabetic community and it will attract more diabetics. Diabetics are significantly more expensive than other patients, even if they get the best possible preventive care.

From an economic point of view, the last thing an HMO wants to do is attract more diabetics. If patients have no choice about belonging to the HMO, then the incentive is to provide the best possible care for diabetics because that care will prevent expensive complications and make these expensive patients less expensive. However, consumer choice (as opposed to just employer choice) is often seen as essential to competition.

Fee for service has a different problem with diabetics. Effective care for diabetics reduces their complications and their need to see the doctor and to have various procedures. Effective diabetic care reduces the income of fee for service providers. For both managed care and fee for service, market competition isn't sending the right kind of signal to induce provider behavior that enhances the value for the diabetic customer. We diabetics have to rely on provider professionalism and ethics to overcome the market incentives.

There is a set of authorities who think competition can be restructured to make it work in the health care marketplace. Prof. Regina Herzlinger of the Harvard Business School presented this view to the NCSL spring meeting in 2003, advocating "consumer driven" health care and the specialization of health care facilities into "focused factories."[6]

Porter and Teisberg are typical of these authorities. They call the current situation "zero sum" competition and acknowledge it isn't working. They think we can move to what they call "positive-sum" competition that will work. They envision a mixture of purchaser (payer) and regulatory changes to force the change. They envision a series of structural modifications with providers aggregating into organizations specializing in particular diseases and becoming quite proficient and efficient in treating those diseases.[7]

There is some evidence that the kind of specialization Herzlinger and Porter and Teisberg envision can work. Porter and Teisberg cite the example of the Texas Heart Institute, which they report specializes in complex and demanding patients but has costs one-third to one-half lower than other academic medical centers.[8] Atul Gawande reports on Shouldice Hospital outside Toronto, Ontario, which specializes in hernia repairs. They have a low recurrence rate and their cost is half what it is elsewhere.[9]

I'm skeptical. There isn't enough specialized volume for their structure to work outside the major metropolitan areas. There are powerful pressures we discussed earlier that can and should keep most health care local. Also, too many patients have several problems at once. Porter and Teisberg acknowledge this problem, but I think their solution (have specialist physicians on staff who can refer to other organizations as needed) is inadequate.

Another problem is the business risks involved in heavy specialization. One risk is governmental. If you specialize in hernias and some bureaucrat in the Department of Health and Human Services (HHS) in Washington (or his provincial equivalent in Toronto in the Shouldice example) decides the reimbursement for doing hernia operations should be reduced, you're in financial trouble. Medicare has a big market share and often Medicaid and even private insurers follow its lead.

A second problem is the risk of scientific advance reducing or wiping out your specialty. Somebody discovers a microorganism is causing the problem that you're treating surgically and suddenly the internists are curing your surgical problem with antibiotics (What happened to the tonsillectomy? What did the discovery of the role of H. Pilori do to the need for ulcer operations?). The protection against these kinds of business risks is larger, less specialized organizations that are diversified in the kinds of work they do.

Another, often overlapping, set of experts advocate "consumer driven" health care. "Consumer driven" seems to mean slightly different things to different people, so you advocates, please forgive me if I don't exactly describe your version of it. A key element of it usually is that the consumer should pay a significant part of the cost out of his own money. The basic idea is that the consumer will be more careful with his own money than some third-party payer's funds.

A simple form of the consumer driven health care system is to have a major increase in deductibles and co-payments with insurance reserved for catastrophic situations. This reduces employers' costs by shifting costs from the employer to the employee. Under current tax law, this can shift health care spending from before tax dollars to after tax dollars, thus reducing the effective compensation the employee gets for any given amount of employer cost. It is happening on quite a scale as employers try to grapple with rising health insurance costs and advocates of consumer health care are seeking to find a tax neutral way of doing it.

Many of the supporters of consumer driven health care are economists who believe in markets as the solution to economic problems. Susan Lee of The Wall Street Journal in an editorial section headed "The Dismal Science" provides a typical example. She recites some of the problems with our health care system including "relentlessly rising costs and bureaucracy" and "profligate use of resources." Then she observes, "Anybody who gives a few hours of thought to the current health care system can identify the mother of these problems — the widespread existence of a third-party payer system." She says the existence of the third-party payer system "insulates consumers of health care from its true cost and encourages overconsumption."

She cites a number of reputable economists who favor changing the tax code to favor insurance with high deductibles and high co-payments. Lee's summary is, "It all makes perfect sense. Since low coinsurance and deductibles are the engine behind rocketing costs and wasteful medical practices, providing consumers with the incentive to shift to policies with high coinsurance and deductibles is an elegant remedy."[10]

The tax problems have led to various plans in which an employer contributes pre-tax dollars to an account which the employee controls. The early version of these was the Medical Savings Account (MSA). The more recent version is the Health Savings Account (HSA), which went into effect January 1, 2004. The HSA is significantly more useful than the MSA because the tax regulations on what can be done with it are significantly more flexible. The specifics of these plans are constrained by the intricacies of the tax laws. What Ms. Lee and the economists she reports on are advocating is a more direct change in the tax laws that doesn't depend on having a special account.

I am skeptical that a "consumer driven" system can have the effects that the supporters envision. There are some practical problems involving incentives for preventive care that possibly can be solved by a careful program design.

More importantly, the majority of health care expenses are in episodes, which are so expensive that the average middle class American either cannot pay for them or cannot do so without debt that threatens bankruptcy.

Such episodes have to be covered by a third-party payer (insurance or government program). A system that does not provide for such coverage will not survive politically. In other words, the assumption that the tax code causes the third-party payer system is a myth. The size and nature of the expenses cause it, and the tax code merely accommodates this reality. In addition, in major illnesses the consumer will figure that preserving life and avoiding disability is more important than money, and either ignore cost, or figure more expensive is better, even if he has to pay a share himself.

Consumer driven health care may save money by giving the consumer an incentive to avoid over-treating minor illnesses and conditions, like ordinary hay fever, where the consequences of inadequate treatment are passing discomfort, not a threat of death or disability. These conditions are not where the big money is.

Let's discuss the practical problems with consumer driven health care first. The various proposals deal with them with varying degrees of success. One of them is that people may skimp on preventive care, saving money in the short run, but costing money in the long run. My observation is that almost everybody is very good at figuring out what his short-term interests are.

I was deeply involved in welfare reform, which was very successful here in Wyoming (90 percent-plus in caseload reduction). A key to our success was we rearranged the benefits so it was in people's short-term financial interest to get off the cash grant welfare system and go to work. We let people keep enough of the benefits (e.g. Medicaid, childcare, food stamps) so they were money ahead to go to work even at a minimum wage job.[11] For a consumer driven health plan, dealing with this short-term incentive problem means delivering useful preventive care that is "free" to the consumer.

Theoretically, this feature should be unnecessary because preventive care is still in people's long-term best interest even if it costs them money in the short term. My observation is that people are less successful at identifying their long-term interests. They're still relatively good at it, but short-term considerations often will trump the long term.

A related problem is that a surprising number of people take a very fatalistic attitude toward the risk of long-term health problems. They see too many examples of people who try hard to do all the right preventive steps and still are unlucky and die early. Too many people just don't understand the idea of statistical improvements in their luck. They figure they've got to die of something someday and that's a matter of luck — in the meantime, they want to eat, drink and be merry and not be bothered. All of us have a little of that attitude. A rich dessert is praised as "sinfully good" and consumed. And how many of you over 50 have had a colonoscopy in the last 10 years?

Consumer driven health plans, being consumer driven, tend to increase these problems, adding an immediate out-of-pocket cost consideration to all the other excuses we have for not getting preventive care that is cost effective in the long term, but costly or unpleasant in the short term.

Another problem is that consumer driven plans usually have some kind of employer-paid incentive for people to hold down costs. Often each month a set amount is put into an account the person controls. If the money is unspent at the end of the year, it can be rebated to the individual, spent on uncovered services, or rolled over to the next year. The problem comes from the people who don't use any care in a given year because they don't need any. They still get the incentives because you have to treat employees alike and you can't tell for sure who at the start of the year is going to need care and who isn't.

The incentive for these people is going to cost the employer (or the government, depending on who is paying) money that will at least partly offset any savings from the consumers being more careful with their health care. The federal government with its tax laws has made at least one of these schemes (the flexible spending account) worse by providing that the amounts in the account expire and revert to the employer at the end of the year, thus providing a use it or lose it incentive.

Another problem is adverse selection. If there's a choice and only the healthy people choose the consumer driven plan, the employer gets the cost of the incentives, but not most of the savings. Halvorson and Isham report that a Health-Partners internal study showed that the people who left its clinics and moved to an MSA (Medical Savings Account) product had much different patterns of preselection care. They averaged half as much cost in care in the year prior to the selection as those who stayed. The incentive was for the healthy people to move while the ones with risks stayed with the traditional plan.

Are the savings enough from those who move to the MSA to overcome the disadvantages of the adverse selection? Again, Halvorson and Isham: "What about the contention that people with an MSA product make better and cheaper care choices? That's very likely true — but statistically irrelevant. If the 70 percent of the population who uses 10 percent of the care buy MSA coverage and become 10 percent more efficient, that cuts the total cost of care by one percent, not exactly a silver bullet."[12]

In this passage Halvorson and Isham have identified what's wrong with consumer driven health care. Even if a whole population, not a self-selected portion of it, is moved to a consumer driven plan, the savings will not be enough to make a big difference.

I have a summary of the distribution of claims for Natrona County School District #1's self-insured plan. More than half of the expenditure came from claims that were greater than $20,000. I suspect this distribution or something close to it is typical. The average employee is not going to be able to afford enough of a share of a $20,000-plus bill to make him a more careful consumer. The "more expensive is better quality" and "go the extra mile to be on the safe side" incentives are going to overwhelm any personal co-payment considerations, especially when the individual is sick and in the hands of doctors he trusts. These considerations will defeat most of the "consumer driven" efforts to use the market to produce the same results in health care that we see elsewhere in the economy.

This is one area of health care where reforms designed to use the free market can produce the kind of beneficial results from competition seen elsewhere in the economy. That is prescription drugs and it is the subject of the next chapter.

Chapter 8, Footnotes

(1) Harvard Business Review, June 2004, editors' summary to "Redefining Competition in Health Care" by Michael E. Porter and Elizabeth Olmstead Teisberg, page 65.

(2) Michael E. Porter and Elizabeth Olmstead Teisberg, "Redefining Competition in Health Care," Harvard Business Review, page 65.

(3) George C. Halvorson & George J. Isham, M.D., Epidemic of Care, Jossye-Bass, 2003. See pages 63-86 and 117-142.

(4) Dr. William Nolen, A Surgeon's World, Fawcett, 1970, pages 116 & 117.

(5) W.S. 26-22-503(a)(iii) and W.S. 26-34-134.

(6) Prof. Regina Herzlinger, Harvard Business School, presentation to NCSL Spring Meeting, Boston, Mass., April 2003.

(7) Porter & Teisberg, Ibid, pages 65-76.

(8) Porter & Teisberg, Ibid, page 67.

(9) Atul Gawande, "Complications, A Surgeon's Notes on an Imperfect Science," Picador, 2002, pages 38-41.

(10) Susan Lee, "A Tax-Code Cure for Ailing Health Care," The Wall Street Journal, August 9, 2004, page A13. Ms. Lee is a member of The Wall Street Journal's editorial board.

(11) I led my committee in drafting our welfare reform legislation (Chapter 111 Session Laws of Wyoming, 1996, passed six months before the national reform legislation and Chapter 196 Session Laws of Wyoming, 1997 adjusting our legislation to the requirements of the national reform). We examined very carefully charts prepared by our Department of Family Services showing how welfare recipients were better off financially under the old system if they did not work and better off working under various new system options. Under the old system, the break-even point where working paid better than not working was surprisingly high (over $9 per hour at a time our statewide average wage was between $10 and $11 an hour). The old welfare system kept people in bondage to the state welfare bureaucracy with a big, short-term incentive to stay on welfare.

(12) Halvorson & Isham, Ibid, pages 184-185.

Chapter 9

PRESCRIPTION DRUGS

In recent years, rising costs for prescription drugs have been an important contributor to rising health care costs. In calculations based on federal data, the Kaiser Family Foundation reported that prescription drugs had risen from 5.8 percent of total health care expenditures in 1990 to 9.4 percent in 2000 and that they accounted for 13.5 percent of the increase in health care costs over that period.[1] The Pricewaterhouse analysis lumped prescription drugs with medical devices and medical advances as 22 percent of the increase in health care premiums for 2001-2002.[2]

It is my theory that effective use of the free market is the way to deal with excessive drug costs. I think governmental actions should be targeted at making the free market effective for prescription drugs. There are some regulatory interventions that can reduce costs for all drug manufacturers, but the best way for these to translate into reduced prices is using a free market mechanism.

Prescription drug costs are not the most important source of rising health care costs. Looking at the decade from 1990 to 2000, Kaiser ranked them fifth with hospital care (26.2 percent of the increase) and physician and clinical services (21.4 percent) being the first and second largest sources of increase,[3] but they are significant, particularly for a couple of key categories of users.

Prescription drug costs are a major problem for many people who are heavy users of prescription drugs and who do not have insurance coverage for those drugs. The majority, but not all, of these people are elderly because the older you are, the more likely you are to need prescriptions and because Medicare until recently had no prescription drug benefit.

I first realized the seriousness of the problem going door to door in my 2000 election campaign. I was asking about people's needs and priorities and encountered many people who either had a problem themselves or had a friend or relative who did. The neighborhoods where I found the most problems were older middle-class neighborhoods with lots of recently retired people. The sense I got was that these people had made reasonable preparations for their retirement — they had paid for low mortgage homes and a pension or reasonable savings to supplement their Social Security.

They thought they had made adequate provisions for a comfortable retirement. Then they were ambushed with $300 to $500-plus a month in prescription drug costs they had not planned for. Drug costs were removing their comfort margin and forcing cutbacks on basics. The drug costs are a major personal problem for these people and a very high percentage of them vote, so they count big time in the politicians' world. This is where the political push came from that finally got a Medicare prescription drug benefit passed in 2003. It will go into full effect in 2006 with a modest start in 2004.

At this writing (fall of 2004), it is not clear to me whether the benefit that goes into effect in 2006 will be a cost effective program and will solve people's problems. The benefit will be delivered by private firms. If these firms have the right incentives, they could deliver a very cost-effective program that will meet people's needs. If they don't, the program could be an expensive mess. The key question is how will those private firms make their money. If we know that, we will know what their incentives are and can predict how they will behave. I have been unable to find any explanation of this key feature and thus cannot predict whether the new program will be a success or a failure.

State budgets are a second place where rising drug costs are causing a major problem. The Medicaid program is the main source of the problem, but state employee insurance benefit costs and health care costs for special populations like the seriously mentally ill and prisoners also are impacted. Medicaid drug costs attract legislators' attention because they aren't costs we can control as directly as most other health costs. If hospital or doctor costs rise in Medicaid, we can hold the line on reimbursements or even cut them back. This may cause problems in the rest of society due to cost shifting, but the immediate impact on the state budget can be controlled.

We eventually may have to increase reimbursements, but we can do it slowly, in response to political pressure, and at a time the state budget can afford it. The Medicaid population will continue to get the service it needs if we are slow to raise reimbursements. Prescription drugs are different. We have to pay the prices that are set by others whether we like it or not. The drug sellers would refuse to provide the drugs if we don't and the federal government would cut off all Medicaid reimbursement for prescription drugs.

Among legislators specializing in health care issues, concern over the budgetary impact of prescription drug costs is being magnified into anger at the drug companies by a rising feeling that they are ripping us off. This concern has been on display at NCSL meetings for the last three or four years — the sessions on drug costs have been well attended and full of angry legislators with hostile questions for the drug company representatives and their allies.

I remember a particular session at the NCSL Health Leaders Seminar in Washington, D.C., in December 2003. A representative from the Food and Drug Administration (FDA) had the job of defending the law banning a popular proposal with many legislators, the re-importation of drugs from Canada and other countries. It didn't help that the FDA representative was making claims about lack of safety of Canadian drugs that most of us in the audience believed were simply untrue. The audience was extremely hostile. I remember thinking at the time that now the FDA man knew how the representatives of King George III must have felt trying to defend the tea duties to hostile colonists in 1775.

Part of the legislative anger stems from the vagaries of drug pricing and the federal restrictions on what the states can do about it. A little history is important here. The prices that states pay for prescription drugs are governed by a federal price control system known as the Medicaid Drug Rebate Program. It was originally enacted as part of the Omnibus Budget Reconciliation Act of 1990 (OBRA 90) and modified in 1993 and 1996. The pricing formula is complicated, but the key provision for most non-generic drugs is a rebate to the states that is based on the manufacturers' best prices and their average wholesale prices in the state in question.[4]

There is a different formula for generic drugs. Drugs used in hospitals and a few other institutional settings are not covered by this rebate system, but are paid for as part of the overall reimbursement to those institutions. Drugs used in outpatient settings, far and away the largest portion of drug usage, are covered. A condition of accepting the rebate is that the state cannot deny access to any drug subject to the rebate, which for practical purposes is all prescription drugs.

The amounts of money involved are significant. Bruen of the Urban Institute reports that for 1998 Medicaid spending for prescription drugs was $14.5 billion after federal and state rebates of $2.5 billion.[5] These rebates come to 14.7 percent of the total original prices. Bruen does not separate the federal rebate program from the smaller state rebate programs, but most of the $2.5 billion must have come from the federal program. The state programs, except for California, were largely started after 1998.

The standard line on the Medicaid drug rebate program is that the feds were trying to help the states keep prescription drug costs down. Bruen reflects this saying, "The federal government set up the Medicaid Drug Rebate Program in 1990 in response to growing concern over the cost of prescription drugs provided to Medicaid patients."[6]

On the face of it, the drug rebate program does look like a standard government health care tactic — a cost increase is causing problems so we will resort to an artificial price control mechanism to hold it down. However, I strongly suspect the law was developed by representatives of the big drug companies, and they knew exactly what they were doing.

In 1990 rising drug prices were starting to hurt and some of the larger states were getting aggressive about demanding volume discounts and using formularies that excluded higher priced drugs. The way a formulary works is that a drug not on the formulary will not be reimbursed and therefore is not used. This is a powerful weapon for a large purchaser who wants a discount, and state actions had the potential of unleashing a price war.

The incentives that are built into the drug rebate formula are a big help to the drug industry. It is a price control mechanism and has the effect a price control usually has — it holds prices up.[7] The effects are felt across the entire prescription drug market, not just the Medicaid program. Suppose a large drug purchaser — say an HMO or a large employer — comes to a drug manufacturer and demands a big volume discount

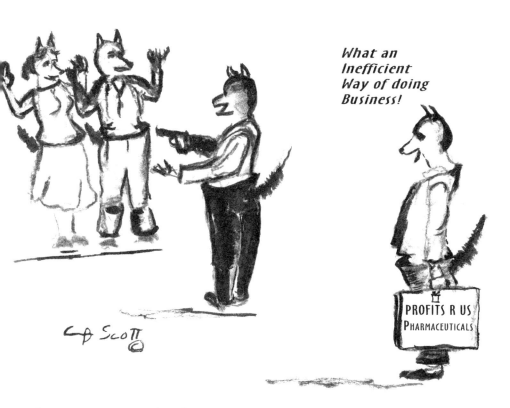

What an
Inefficient
Way of doing
Business!

PROFITS R US
PHARMACEUTICALS

threatening to take their business elsewhere if they don't get
it. The drug company has to say, "Can't do it. If I give you a discount beyond the 15.1 percent mandatory state rebate, I have
to give the same to the state Medicaid program in the form of
an additional rebate. That's the law. I can't get out of it.' Medicaid's a big purchaser; you can't supply enough volume to
make up for that rebate." Because the law is the same for
everyone, the other drug companies will say the same thing.

The initial drug company pricing structure builds in some
level of discount for all the large purchasers, including the
Medicaid program. They need to keep some level of rebate to
prevent the states from abandoning the federal rebate program. They have to give a minimum rebate of at least 15.1 percent from the average price (AMP) so there is some room for
volume discounting before the size of the rebate is affected.

The net effect is that the people who pay the highest price
are the retail customers not covered by insurance — the
people too poor to afford insurance with a good drug benefit
and the senior citizens on Medicare paying their own bills.

Our health care system has a proclivity for sticking those who can least afford it with the highest prices. The government is often, as in this case, responsible and frequently in cahoots with major providers.

The formula contains an additional incentive for the drug companies to set the initial prices of drugs high. Price increases for drugs are limited to the general CPI increase. Higher increases lead to additional rebates. If a drug company makes a mistake and prices a drug too low for market conditions or too low to recover all the costs (like legal expenses if there is an unforeseen side effect or manufacturing costs if there are problems scaling up production and unexpected costs there), the formula would appear not to allow the mistake to be rectified. It's far better to price on the high side and back down as conditions dictate.

The incentives in the rebate system are legal, work uniformly across the industry, and are much more effective than any illegal conspiracy in restraint of trade in preventing price competition in prescription drugs.

The "best price" provision in the formula is another source of state anger over prescription drug pricing. The feds exempted themselves from the best price calculation with the result that several large health care providers that are active in our communities, including the VA and the federally qualified health centers, get prices that are much below what the state can get.

Another source of problems with the rebate system is the secrecy it requires. Federal law forbids the states to reveal the net prices after rebates we actually pay for prescription drugs. We can report aggregate spending and break it down by category, but we cannot reveal the net price we pay for an individual drug. We can't tell our citizens how much a month's supply of a particular drug costs us. I know of no other major expenditures where the state cannot make public the unit prices we pay for items we purchase.

The federal secrecy requirement is a problem for state prescription drug reform efforts because it prevents states from communicating with citizens as effectively as desired. We can't use the kinds of examples of savings for specific drugs we would like to. As one author, writing about the Oregon plan said, "The cost-effectiveness process cannot be fully disclosed because of federal Medicaid law regarding rebates and pricing of Medicaid drug purchases. This threatens the public credibility of the process."[8]

A practical effect of the federal secrecy requirement is that it precludes effective auditing of the rebate system. The federal law is so restrictive that knowledge of the rebates and thus the net prices paid are restricted to the employees of the Medicaid agency. This means we cannot use either hired outside auditors or even the state audit agency for an audit of the system. My experience is that complex financial systems tend to drift out of compliance in favor of whoever makes the actual computations unless subjected to regular audit. There is too much incentive to shade anything that might be a gray area. The Medicaid Drug Rebate Program is certainly a complex financial system, and it is the drug companies that calculate the rebates and make the payments.

There are several proposals for reform to deal with the problem of rising prescription drug costs. To understand these it is necessary to first take a quick look at the economic basics causing the drug companies to price their products the way they do.

In general, prescription drugs are characterized by high up front costs for R&D and for obtaining regulatory approval. The numbers are large, the industry reports spending $31 billion on R&D in 2002.[9] Cutler pegs the cost of developing the average new drug at $500 million including the costs of testing (for regulatory approval?) and paying for the failures.[10] These costs do not vary with the volume sold except for some regulatory breaks for so called "orphan drugs," which help rare conditions and can't generate enough sales to justify the costs of full regulatory approval.

Promotional and marketing expenses are the next big category of drug expenses with the industry reporting $21 billion spending in 2002.[11] This spending is not a fixed cost. It is discretionary and should cause an increase in the volumes of marketed drugs sold, but it does not go up automatically with unit volume. Usually the costs to manufacture the drug and to distribute it to patients are relatively small, and those costs should vary directly with volume. The economics of the drug industry therefore involve high fixed costs and low variable costs.

Under these circumstances, if there is a market where the fixed costs can be recovered through high unit prices, greatly discounted prices can be allowed in subordinate markets, provided the discounts don't spread to the main markets. A greatly discounted price, provided it is above the directly variable costs (i.e. the manufacturing and distribution costs), still will make some contribution to fixed costs and thus profits. If, however, the discounts spread too much to the main market, the fixed costs will no longer be recovered and the business becomes unprofitable.

The AIDS drugs provide an example. They are sold at high prices in the United States. Most of the fixed costs are recovered and the profits made in this market. We are wealthy and we can afford it. They are sold at vastly discounted prices in Africa, which is a poor country and cannot afford the full price. But if the African prices are at all above manufacturing and distribution costs, it still pays the drug companies to sell there. This pricing structure takes from each market in accord with its ability to pay and, hopefully, provides each market in accord with its needs.

This sounds quite Marxist, but, for a product with the cost structure that prescription drugs have, it makes good free market sense. I know this is an idealized picture of the markets and there are problems of pricing and affordability in both the American and African markets, but these problems do not change the economic principles involved.

A byproduct of this pricing structure is that the drug companies will concentrate on developing drugs for the American market and concentrate on getting regulatory approval here first. Then they can bring the drug to market here first and maximize the amount of time to recover fixed costs and make profits in this market before the patent runs out.

It is in our interest for both humanitarian and economic reasons to see that deeply discounted pricing structures for drugs are maintained in poor Third World countries. If drugs from their markets leak back into the United States, the drug companies will have to raise prices there or stop selling. Either result will deprive the people in those countries of drugs they need and hurt us economically by removing what little contribution to fixed costs they are making.

The developed countries like Canada and Europe are a different matter. In those markets, if the price goes up, it will be paid. People will not be deprived of drugs. They (or their government) can afford the higher prices. In those countries, government price controls often have kept the price of drugs artificially low. The drug manufacturers have tolerated this because the U.S. market remains the one where they recover the bulk of their fixed costs. For us, however, it means that the rest of the developed world is getting a free ride at our expense. If we can encourage smuggling of drugs from those countries, eventually the prices there will have to go up and our prices should come down and there will be a fairer distribution of paying for the R&D costs.

This is what the drug "re-importation" row is all about. The drug companies want to discourage importation from elsewhere as it threatens their high prices here and they have enlisted the federal government to help them. It is a turf issue with the FDA which wants sole governmental responsibility for assuring safety and does not want to rely on any foreign government. It's probably mostly a matter of campaign contributions with the Congress. I think if the federal government was really looking out for our national interest, it would encourage "re-importation." I put "re-importation" in quotes because the drugs often are manufactured not in the U.S. but some third country (e.g. Ireland) and imported into both the U.S. and the "re-importation" source like Canada.

How should the individual react to an opportunity to obtain drugs abroad? When dealing with sources in Canada or Britain or any other country where there are effective drug safety laws and governmental corruption is unusual, the safety concerns should be no greater than for similar sources in the U.S. I would recommend a little care to make sure any Internet or mail order sources are reputable. In countries where there is significant governmental corruption or inadequate drug regulation, I would be much more wary. One way for a dishonest operator to make money is to sell fake drugs to the gringos and pay off the relevant government inspectors.

With this caution, go for it if it pays for you. By "re-importing" drugs, you will be saving yourself money, helping our country economically and resisting silly governmental regulations, all virtuous activities. If you violate some federal regulations in the process, you will be joining the great smuggling tradition that helped the original 13 colonies down the road to independence. How many of our founding fathers and their political allies were involved in smuggling to avoid British tariffs?

For both practical and ethical reasons, I would not re-import drugs from Third World countries. They cannot have the same degree of safety policing of their drug supply that we have because they cannot afford it. In addition, re-importation will threaten their price discounts and may deprive their citizens of access to needed drugs.

I doubt that through re-importation and the other trade agreement efforts our government is making we will ever be able to achieve drug pricing parity with the rest of the developed world. We should be able to narrow the difference to make smuggling less economically attractive, being the market where full costs are recovered does bring us significant advantages. There is an incentive to bring the drugs to market in the U.S. first, so we get the benefit of advances first. In addition, our pricing policies have caused drug companies to concentrate their R&D operations in the U.S. These are high quality, good paying jobs and a major boost to our economy.

One solution to our high drug costs that we should resist is formal price regulation. Recovery of the high costs of R&D, including the risk of failure, is essential in some markets and ours is that market. If we went to a formal price regulation, we could lower our drug costs in the short term, but the price would be likely to be killing off the incentives for the research effort required to develop new drugs. It is in the interest of each of us who wants the longest and healthiest life possible to avoid killing off this research effort. We are not some minor European country like France or Germany who can cut back their drug R&D effort to save money, knowing the United States will pick up the slack.

Regulation of some of the other drug company costs is a different matter. It is useful to periodically review the FDA drug approval practices to make sure they are not unreasonably costly. There always will be a debatable line between the costly studies needed to assure safety and efficacy of a new drug and those required because some mid-level staffer is curious or is throwing his weight around to make a big corporation jump. I think a periodic, critical review of FDA requirements by outside disinterested parties concerned about both cost and safety is indicated.

Curbing litigation excesses is another area where action may be needed. Effective drugs have to be powerful and therefore have risks of side effects. For most of the population, the risks should greatly outweigh the benefits. If they do not, then the FDA should not let the drug on the market. For the person hit by the rare side effect, however, the damage can be considerable. The FDA tries to deal with this problem by identifying the potential side effects and getting doctors to recognize the start of them and take action before significant harm is done. Sometimes the rarer side effects are not found in the FDA safety trials and show up only after widespread use. The costs in both money and time to completely remove this risk are excessive. Bluntly speaking, we will kill more people by delaying getting the product on the market than we will save by taking the time to find every small risk.

So far we are living with the litigation risks although we have had to introduce a no-fault compensation system for vaccine side effects because we were losing our vaccine manufacturers. I think there is a very real chance we should take steps to curb litigation over prescription drug safety so it does not kill off the effort to develop new drugs. I would like to see a careful objective analysis of what litigation is doing to our drug costs. It may already exist, but I have not found it.

Another area where regulation may be in order is marketing and promotion. If we can uniformly remove a marketing cost for all prescription drugs, maybe we should do it. Again, by cutting the costs, we should be able to reduce prices, especially if we adopt a cost control strategy that emphasizes free market competition.

Direct-to-consumer advertising like the TV adds we all see is one such cost. If one company advertises its products directly to the consumer, there is tremendous pressure for all to do so to protect their market shares. If the government forbids such advertising, we may be able to bring down the costs for all, reducing prices.

It is possible that advertising does influence people to take needed medications (e.g. blood pressure medicines), but this is offset because it can induce some people to take unnecessary medication and others to switch from cheap but effective generics to more expensive brand names (especially in blood pressure medications where a federal study showed the generic diuretic was the most effective single medication for most people).

Anecdotally, I hear a common response of doctors in our litigious society is to take the attitude that the customer is always right and to give people asking for an advertised drug what they want. They do it even if it may be unnecessary or more expensive or in the long run, an adequate, but not the best, choice. As a practical matter, direct-to-consumer advertising has to be regulated nationally, so this is a matter for the Congress to consider.

The effort to promote drugs to doctors is another area where we could reduce costs for all companies. Some of this effort is necessary — a drug company with a new product has to get the word to doctors (and other prescribers) that their product exists or it will not be prescribed. As I pointed out in Chapter 5, the excessive time a new innovation takes to become standard practice is a real problem for American medicine. And drug company efforts to promote their drugs can shorten this time for their innovations.

Some of the promotion efforts like free pens and notepads are relatively cheap, harmless and common across American business. Free samples can be very useful for a doctor trying a patient on a new medicine or taking care of a patient with economic problems. They also can steer a patient to an unnecessarily expensive choice A possible reform is to require price information to accompany the free sample.

A free meal may be a reasonable price to pay to get a doctor to pay attention long enough to hear a professional pitch on the advantages (and risks and side effects) of a new drug. However, there is the possibility of excesses, particularly if the doctor is getting some reward for the volume of prescriptions he writes for a particular drug. This represents a conflict of interest and should be guarded against and prohibited.

In veterinary medicine, the vets often sell the medicines they recommend. As a rancher I sometimes am skeptical of their recommendations because I know they make money personally by selling the drugs they recommend. I do not want to see this practice spread to human medicine. There are effective protections against doing it directly, but the problem may be coming in the back door with certain promotional activities. Unlike direct-to-consumer advertising, this is something that states can regulate directly, and I think we should examine the possibilities. It is possible that with some reasonable standards and limits, we can prevent conflicts of interest and reduce drug costs by reducing promotion expenses. We will have to be careful because we don't want to go too far and slow down the adoption of new drugs that really are an improvement. It will require some experimentation, and that's something the states can do successfully.

The states are seeking ways around the federal price control system in Medicaid and are making some progress. Florida, Oregon and Michigan have programs that are being copied elsewhere. There are significant differences between the programs, but all depend on the right that the state has under the OBRA 93 amendments to require prior authorization to dispense a particular drug. The state establishes a preferred drug list made up of the least expensive or most effective drugs in every class. These drugs can be prescribed without further approval. The other drugs in the class are available, but require prior approval.

Often, manufacturers can get their drug added to the preferred drug list if they are willing to meet the price of the drug already on the list, the so-called reference drug. The mechanism used is called a supplemental rebate, but it really amounts to traditional price competition via a discount.

A model for many of the states has been the British Columbia Reference Drug Program. An excellent evaluation of that program was published in the May/June 2004 Health Affairs. I have not found information as comprehensive on the various state programs, probably partly because they have been operating for less time and partly because the federal secrecy requirements inhibit the use of specific savings examples that are available in British Columbia. Under the B.C. program, the Therapeutics Initiative (TI) at the University of British Columbia reviews individual drugs for evidence that they are more effective than cheaper existing drugs.

To quote Health Affairs, "For each drug class considered, the TI was asked to determine whether scientifically valid evidence indicated the superiority of any drug in terms of morbidity or mortality. In the absence of such evidence, PharmaCare [the B.C. public program] based its public subsidy on low cost options within the class."[12] One caution is that because it demands superiority in terms of morbidity or mortality, the B.C. system is skeptical when the evidence is of improved indicators.

Lowering bad cholesterol would be an indicator; fewer fatal heart attacks would be superiority in mortality. Since for a chronic condition evidence of an improved indicator is likely to be available before evidence of the ultimate outcome, this B.C. practice can be expected to slow down the adoption of new drugs that are real improvements.

Currently TI is doing some work on whole drug classes, but mostly they review individual drugs for evidence they are superior to existing choices. Such reviews are easier to do than whole class reviews.[13]

The savings from the British Columbia program have been major. The initial review, released in 1994, was of nitrate drugs used to treat stable angina. B.C. PharmaCare was spending $ 3.8 million per year on a slow-release nitroglycerin product that costs 10 times as much per usual dose as the alternatives. The TI review found no evidence in existing literature that the slow-release product had an advantage in efficacy, effectiveness, compliance, or side effects.[14]

The new Cyclooxygenase-2 (COX-2) inhibitors, used to treat arthritis, provide another example. COX-2 inhibitors compete with older NSAIDs (Nonsteroidal Anti-Inflammatory Drugs) like ibuprofen and naproxen, but are more expensive. The TI review found the relative safety and efficacy were unknown. There was some evidence of sub-clinical advantages, so in August 2000 PharmaCare required patients to try three other NSAIDs before COX-2 inhibitors would be publicly subsidized. This restricted status was maintained following a scientific scandal over a misleading published report on the comparative therapeutic value of one of the COX-2 inhibitors.[15] The report, which was the subject of U.S. FDA public hearings, disclosed only an early portion of two trials when the full length of the trials revealed more serious side effects that led TI to conclude the data suggested the two COX-2 inhibitors had "a net safety disadvantage in overall patient health."[16]

The savings from B.C.'s restrictions are major. In Ontario, provincial spending on COX-2 inhibitors and other NSAIDs in 2002 was $50 per senior; B.C. PharmaCare spent less than $7 for a net savings to PharmaCare of $23 million.[17]

The drug industry naturally does not like the PharmaCare Reference Drug Program. In the COX-2 case, the Health Affairs article reports it costs the manufacturers $40 million annually in sales. Opposition has included "legal challenges, negative media campaigns, and threats to cease drug industry funding of research in British Columbia."[18] From discussions with other legislators, I predict any state starting a similar program can expect similar drug industry opposition starting with hordes of lobbyists if legislation is required. Sell it to the other legislators as economic development for the capital city hotel/restaurant industry.

The B.C. program has saved the taxpayers money without harming patients. To quote the Health Affairs article, "Furthermore, with special exemptions put in place to deal with patients' idiosyncratic needs and options for patients to use their own funds to purchase products that do not meet the criteria for outcomes-based coverage, these savings have not come with adverse effects associated with indiscriminate cost-shifting policies."

This same article also suggests a spillover effect in the private sector with PharmaCare coverage policies altering the prescribing patterns for private pay patients (the majority in B.C.). Per capita spending on prescription drugs in B.C. grew by 84 percent from 1993 to 2002 while in the rest of Canada, it grew by 104 percent in the same period.[19]

I happened to be at a meeting with some senior people from British Columbia's program the day after Merck withdrew Vioxx, its widely-used Cox-2 inhibitor, from the market due to safety concerns. The B.C. people's attitude was best described as vindicated rather than smug. They had taken a lot of heat over their restrictions on Cox-2 inhibitors, and Merck's action showed their restrictions were justified.

It may also be that British Columbia was correct in allowing some limited access to Cox-2 inhibitors including Vioxx. There are people for whom a Cox-2 inhibitor may be a better choice than the standard over-the-counter remedies because these remedies can have adverse side effects with long-term regular use. It may even be that for some people Vioxx is the best choice. That depends on whether other Cox-2 drugs work for them (and are found to be .safer) .It also depends on the relative risks posed for them by the over-the-counter remedies compared to the risks of Vioxx. I have not seen an analysis of these relative risks for this population. I am afraid we may not get it; the final decision on Vioxx may depend more on hype, emotion and the risk of litigation than an objective analysis of its risks compared to those of other alternatives. Sometimes in this world the real choice is not between safe and unsafe. It is between risky and more risky, and our society does not seem to deal with this reality well.

There are some differences among the states in the kinds of pre-authorization programs they have. Florida cut a deal with Pfizer for disease management services expected to save $30 million a year in return for including Pfizer drugs on its preferred list. Michigan does not allow this and used a state-appointed panel of pharmacists and physicians to evaluate drugs based on clinical effectiveness, safety, outcomes and cost, and to chose at least "two best in class" drugs in 40 different classes.[20] As is required by federal Medicaid regulations, physicians can get authorization for drugs not on the preferred list for patients who need them, but in Michigan this is a relatively difficult bureaucratic process. In Oregon, possibly because Rep. Al Bates, M.D., helped write the legislation, it is quite easy for the physician to override the preferred drug list and get a non-preferred drug authorized.

Oregon uses a more public process for choosing the preferred drugs and is doing outcomes research similar to British Columbia's. A number of other states, including Wyoming, have paid to subscribe to (and thereby support) Oregon's research efforts. There is an informal professional cooperation between Oregon and British Columbia — they are doing similar work and the effect of drugs on people does not change with the international border even if the prices do. Oregon's work is currently more focused on reviews of whole classes. Both Oregon and British Columbia are using Cochrane Collaboration standards and methods in their reviews.[21]

It is still too early to get a comprehensive understanding of how much the preferred drug lists will save the states. Many of the programs were delayed by litigation, a common tactic of the drug manufacturers. The program design does make a difference. Oregon's public process for selecting the list was slower than Michigan's, and it is easier for a physician to override the preferred status and prescribe a non-preferred alternative, both of which should diminish Oregon's savings compared to Michigan's.

The pharmaceutical industry has denounced state preferred drugs lists and the accompanying demand for supplemental rebates (discounts) as a price control mechanism. Nothing could be further from the truth. Preferred drug lists are a mechanism for market competition. In most classes of drugs there are multiple drugs available that do the same thing. Sometimes there are differences in how well the drugs do and usually there are differences in price. This is the circumstance where we should expect market competition to reward the best combination of efficacy and price.

This is the opportunity for competition to push value in drugs as it has in other parts of the economy like computers or automobiles. So far it hasn't either because the purchasers lack the knowledge of the relative quality and prices or because they lack the motivation. By focusing purchasing on some combination of efficacy and price, the preferred drug lists focus the competition on value, at least where the state government is paying the bill. My reading is that the drug companies don't like to be subject to real marketplace competition because it will put at risk the profits of those who don't keep up with the competition.

In Wyoming, we are trying a different tactic based on the same theme. We are working on a preferred drug list, but we also are trying to improve private purchasing directly. Preferred drug lists help only Medicaid and other state programs directly. They have no direct effect on private purchases although there may be an indirect spillover effect in the private sector as appears to have happened in British Columbia.

In August 2002, my legislative committee held a public hearing on rising health care costs and what should be done about them. We invited people with ideas to come talk to us. One of those we heard from was Ralph Bartholomew, a pharmacist who worked for one of our major employers trying to hold down its prescription drug costs and also did volunteer work for his local senior citizens' center. He reviewed individual patient's drug prescriptions and achieved major savings by getting people to substitute cheaper drugs that were just as effective. He had his clients check his recommendations with their doctor. This is a regulatory requirement and a sensible one.

Occasionally the patient's doctor would have a specific reason why that patient should not be switched, but

Bartholomew's testimony was the reason that doctors approved his recommendations more than 90 percent of the time. We thought this sounded sensible so we instituted a program where the state would pay for this kind of consultation for any citizen who wanted it.[22] Any Wyoming citizen can request the consultation by calling a toll-free number (1-877-246-4114). There is a $75 consultation fee of which the state pays $70 and the individual $5. The University of Wyoming's School of Pharmacy runs the program under contract from our Health Department.

In its brochure promoting this program, Wyoming AARP cited an example of one of its members who saved $85 a month or $1,020 annually through this consultation. For this person the pharmacist found a $12 per month drug that could be substituted for a $43 a month one and recommended the person phase out another medicine costing $29 per month. The pharmacist also discovered the person was taking too many vitamins and got a $25 a month savings from eliminating the excess.[23] This particular consultation had more savings from elimination of unneeded drugs and less from substitution of cheaper drugs than some and saved less than average. Through May of 2004, the average savings per consultation was $1,700 per year.

The combination of third-party payers using evidence-based formularies, preferred drug lists and pharmacist consultations for individual purchasers is an effective way to use the free market to control drug costs. As this system takes hold, drug companies will have to be price competitive in drug classes where there are multiple products that do mostly the same thing. When they have a significantly better product and a new breakthrough that really has better outcomes, they will be able to charge much higher prices. That will be expensive for anyone needing the new product, but worth it.

Under this system, the market will be sending the correct signal to the drug companies — there will be financial rewards for new products that are better. They should invest in the R&D to find such products. For the others, they have to improve value by holding down prices. It will be unsafe for companies to rest on their laurels and push knock-offs of other products. The market will demand improvement and continuously ask, "What have you done for me lately?"

Chapter 9, Footnotes

(1) The Henry J. Kaiser Family Foundation, Trends and Indicators in the Changing Health Care Marketplace, 2002, Chartbook May 2002. he Kaiser staff made calculations based on data from the Centers for Medicaid and Medicare Services (CMS), Office of the Actuary, National Health Statistics Group.

(2) PriceWaterhouseCoopers, "The Factors Fueling Rising Healthcare Costs," April 2002, analysis prepared for the American Association of Health Plans, pages 3-5. See also appendix 2 of this book.

(3) Kaiser, Ibid, page 11.

(4) Brian K. Bruen, The Urban Institute, Washington, D.C., "Medicaid and Prescription Drugs: An Overview," prepared for and published by the Kaiser Commission on Medicaid and the Uninsured, The Henry J. Kaiser Family Foundation, page 4. The paper reports the formula for the so-called "innovator products" (non-generic drugs) is "(1) a rebate that is the greater of 15.1 percent of the average manufacturer's price (AMP) per unit or the difference between the AMP and the manufacturer's 'best price' per unit, and (2) an additional rebate for any price increase for a product that exceeds the increase in the Consumer Price Index (CPI-U) for all items since the fall of 1990. The AMP is the average price paid by wholesalers in the state for products distributed to the retail pharmacy class of trade. The best price is the lowest price offered any other customer, excluding Federal Supply Schedule prices, prices to state pharmaceutical assistance programs, and prices that are nominal in amount."

(5) Bruen, Ibid, page 5.

(6) Bruen, Ibid, page 5.

(7) I will confess I am particularly skeptical about the value of price controls due to my personal experience. In 1974 I quit the federal government in Washington, D.C., and came back to Wyoming to run the family cattle ranch. In the fall of 1973, cattle prices were high, restricted by President Nixon's price controls designed to fight inflation. In 1974 the price controls came off and the prices of cattle collapsed. We got 74 cents a pound for our calves in the fall of 1973 and 33 cents in the fall of 1974. A 400-pound calf was worth more per animal in 1993 than the same animal was worth as a 750-pound yearling a year later. The price controls had hurt both the consumer and the producer by masking the price signals that the marketplace should have been sending. For me, it was a rough introduction to the cattle business.

(8) Draft RSG (Reforming States Group) Discussion Paper on Prescription Drug Costs and Access 10/30/2002, page 19.

(9) "Rx Update," June 2004, a publication of the Pharmaceutical Research and Manufacturers of America, citing PhRMA Annual Membership survey, 2004.

(10) David M. Cutler, <u>Your Money or Your Life, Strong Medicine for America's Health Care System</u>, Oxford University Press, 2004, page 83. Cutler's source is cited as Joseph DiMasi et al., "The Cost of Innovation in the Pharmaceutical Industry," Journal of Health Economics, Vol. 10 No. 2 (July 1991), pages 107-142. It is not clear whether Cutler has adjusted the number for inflation since 1991, so even the $500 million per drug figure could be significantly too low.

(11) "Rx Update, "Ibid," citing IMS Health, "Integrated Promotional Services, tm" and CMR, 2/2003.

(12) Steven Morgan, Ken Bassett and Barbara Mintzes, "Outcomes-Based Drug Coverage in British Columbia," Health Affairs, Vol. 23, No. 3, May/June 2004, page 271.

(13) Author's conversation with Robert Nakagawa, director of Pharmacy, Fraser Health Authority, British Columbia, July 6, 2004.

(14) Morgan et al., Ibid, page 271.

(15) F.E. Silverstein et al., "Gastrointestinal Toxicity with Celecoxib vs. Nonsteroidal Anti-Inflammatory Drugs for Osteoarthritis and Rheumatoid Arthritis; The CLASS Study: A Randomized Controlled Trial," Journal of the American Medical Association, 286, No. 10 (2000), pages 1247-1255.

(16) Morgan et al., Ibid, page 272.

(17) Morgan et al., Ibid, page 273. It is not clear from the article whether these are U.S. or Canadian dollars.

(18) Morgan et al., Ibid, page 273 (sales figures) and 272 (quotation).

(19) Morgan et al., Ibid, page 274.

(20) National Conference of State Legislators, "State Health Lawmakers' Digest," Vol. 2, No. 3, Spring 2002.

(21) Author's conversation with Robert Nakagawa, July 6, 2004.

(22) Chapter 85, Session Laws of Wyoming, 2003, W.S. 9-2-124.

(23) Brochure entitled "Safe effective ways to SAVE on your pharmacy bills," published by AARP Wyoming, 2004.

Chapter 10

WORKFORCE ISSUES

This chapter will explore issues about both the cost and the supply of our health workforce that affect the availability, price and quality of our health care. We will start with the cost issues first and then go on to the supply, but of course when the supply is tight, the cost can be expected to go up.

A number of authorities have identified provider prices as a major reason, even the most important reason, why health care is more expensive here in America than in the rest of the world. An article in Health Affairs entitled "It's the Prices Stupid: Why the United States Is So Different From Other Countries," is typical. It says, "The data show that the United States spends more on health care than any other country. However, on most measures of health services use, the United States is below the OECD median. These facts suggest that the difference in spending is caused mostly by higher prices for health care goods and services in the United States."[1]

The article acknowledges the role of our excessive administrative costs in our higher prices and recognizes the special cases of prescription drugs and high tech devices. It does not recognize the litigation risk premium built into our prices, but this factor is there even if not quantified. It spends considerable time analyzing the roles of monopoly and monopsony power on both the purchaser and provider sides.

The analysis of monopoly and monopsony effect is interesting, especially if you like economic theory, but is somewhat beside the point. The basics are fairly clear. Health care is labor intensive, especially in its use of skilled professional labor. For example, a study done for The BlueCross BlueShield Association reported that workforce costs represent 50 percent of a hospital's operating expense. Nurse cost center direct costs which are 80 percent payroll are 44 percent of hospital inpatient costs.[2] Our modern society pays skilled professional labor very well. This is true in all the developed countries, but it is especially true in the United States.

Our labor market is especially free and that has resulted in good pay for skilled professionals. If we don't pay nurses and various bachelor's and master's degree-level professionals well, they will quit and earn more (or enjoy better working conditions if that is the issue) doing something else. Someone who has the intelligence and scientific education to enter one of these professions has the ability to do a wide range of other things and do them well.

In our free labor market people can and will switch out of health care if it is in their interest to do so. The result is shortages which result in higher prices. The BlueCross BlueShield report stated that each one percent increase in the RN shortage at the state level was associated with a 0.96 percent increase in hospital inpatient costs per member of a large health plan.[3] I think it is this factor more than any considerations of provider monopoly pricing power that drives what our health care providers charge.

The case is a little less clear with medical doctors. There are fewer competing occupations in which a doctor can enter and have earnings that can exceed what they can earn as a medical doctor. There are some who have left medicine for business, law or other careers. Medical fees are set more by tradition, intensity of the care given and length of post-M.D. training required than by market forces. The market influence is more indirect — if doctors' incomes are not excellent, fewer of the best and the brightest will be willing to enter the lengthy and expensive training required to be a doctor.

Once the training is finished, the doctor has made a big investment in time and money and has foregone many of the opportunities to enter a competing high compensation occupation. The existing doctor population can be squeezed provided you don't care about the resulting effect on our ability to recruit the best into the profession. However, any strategy of controlling costs by squeezing the doctors too hard runs the risk of driving some of them to other occupations.

We are widely believed to have shortages of most of the health care occupations. A report published by the Milbank Memorial Fund states the conventional wisdom well: "For a variety of reasons, most regions of the nation are experiencing shortages in an array of health professions." And the problem is expected to get worse. To quote the same report,

"The Bureau of Labor Statistics (BLS) in the U.S. Department of Labor has projected that the number of health care jobs will grow nearly 20 percent between 2000 and 2010. This is twice the rate of growth of jobs in the rest of the economy."

The reasons are partly demographic and partly due to our growing technical abilities. Again the Milbank Report, "In any case, continued long-term growth in the health sector, combined with an aging population and an aging health workforce will create a major challenge for the nation during the next 30 years."[4]

The nursing shortage is one that has attracted a lot of attention. Most states currently have a shortage of nurses and that shortage is expected to grow as the baby boomer generation ages and needs more health care. Yet the supply of new nurses is contracting. End-of-life care expert Joanne Lynn citing the National Council of State Boards of Nursing reports that the number of first-time U.S.-educated nursing school graduates who sat for the national licensure examination for registered nurses fell by 25 percent from 1995 to 2002.[5] It is not clear the extent to which this decline is caused by a drop in academic training opportunities and to what extent to a decline in the numbers of prospective students due to problems with wages, hours and working conditions.

Hours and working conditions are important in the nursing shortages. Hospital nursing of absolute necessity involves shift work, which is unpopular. In the individual setting, how the nurses are treated is very important. When the doctors and the patients treat nurses like the skilled professional members of the team that they are, the nurses will be much happier with their work than when they are treated like servants, which also can happen.

The obvious solution to shortages of health care professionals is to expand the training opportunities for new ones. This is a slow process. It takes a minimum of seven years after college to train a doctor (four years medical school plus three years of residency). Expanding a medical school takes some planning time, and creating a new one takes even more time. The same is true for other health professions although the times are less.

The cost of training new health care professionals is a major problem. They are more expensive to train than most other professions. They need expensive laboratory space, and opportunities for clinical experience. The faculty is more expensive than other university faculty. The university has to pay higher salaries because otherwise the instructors will leave the university for positions practicing the profession. In addition to finding the money in a time of tight budgets, this necessity for higher pay causes jealousy among the faculty in the less lucrative fields.

In addition to the budgetary and faculty pay problems, expanding health professional training can run into opposition from an instinctive academic resistance to change due to real world pressures. The net effect is that academic institutions sometimes resist pressure to expand health professional training. In the Wyoming Legislature, we hit this problem in 2003 when we passed legislation to expand the training of nurses. We proposed an incentive to expand enrollments in nursing programs and the University of Wyoming was not interested in participating. Fortunately our community colleges were. We wrote the university out of the expansion part of the legislation and restricted the incentives for expansion to the community colleges.[6]

Expanding the training opportunities is only one part of the equation in getting new people into the health care workforce. Persuading people to take advantage of the opportunities is another part. In Wyoming we have been able to fill our expanded nursing education slots, but I have heard anecdotally that this is not always the case in the rest of the country. Nursing and other health professions have to compete with other opportunities for the best people. As discussed before, pay and working conditions are important. Young adults' perceptions of the profession and its social status is important as well.

The time and difficulty of expanding training opportunities means that in the short term, other steps are going to be needed to meet our health manpower shortages. One of these is pay. The marketplace will respond to shortages by demanding and getting higher pay. To some extent, increases in pay will just shift the shortage from those institutions and locations raising pay to those not doing so, forcing them to match the increases. However as pay increases, people who have left the profession will return increasing supply. There also will be increasing pressure from students for more training opportunities. Money talks. The implication is that pay raises are going to be a source of increased health care costs for some time.

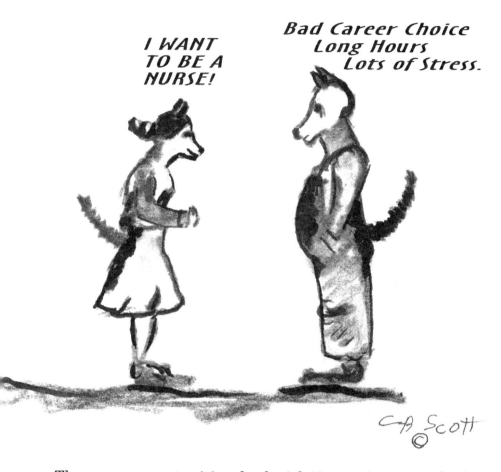

There are opportunities for legislative action to make it easier for people to come back into a health care profession. The problems that need to be solved are often in the licensure area. While they are out of the profession, people let their licenses lapse or lose them due to failure to keep up with the continuing education requirements. My experience is that the various health care professions and the several states vary wildly in how hard it is for someone to rejoin a profession.

If a state is having a shortage of a particular health professional, one of the first places I would look is how hard is it to bring back someone who has left the profession and is willing to return. In some cases, modifications to the law will be indicated; in others the executive branch needs to appoint different people to licensing boards to get ones who are less rigid guardians of professional purity. One technique to consider, particularly if a profession has undergone considerable change in recent years, is a provisional license with a requirement for a period of mentoring or refresher courses, or both.

Another area that should be looked at is licensing reciprocity. As our society becomes more mobile, professionals are moving more often, sometimes following a spouse. Many of the health professions have the process of getting licenses by reciprocity well thought out and appropriately easy, but this is not universally true. Sometimes legislative change is needed.

Another tactic for dealing with a shortage of professionals is to turn some of a profession's functions over to a profession which requires less training or even develop such a profession. This is very common and sometimes is quite contentious.

The history of most health professions is a drive to improve the education and training of the profession coupled with an expansion of what the profession can do. For medical doctors the expansion has come from the expansion of our scientific knowledge and ability to diagnose and treat. In most of the other professions, at least some of the expansion has come from an invasion of turf that once exclusively belonged to another profession, often medicine.

Take physical therapy. The profession started as an adjunct to the physician in treating crippling diseases like polio and strokes. Physicians diagnosed the problems, decided what therapy was needed, and the physical therapist gave the patient the treatment. The preparation required was a bachelor's degree. From the beginning, the therapist had a role in determining the exact nature of the exercises or other therapy required, but the physician had close supervision of what was done. Gradually the therapists learned more about techniques for evaluating symptoms of the diseases and conditions they were treating.

This knowledge enabled them to do a better job providing therapy. Therapists began doing independent evaluations of patients, first to help design therapy programs and then to provide independent diagnoses (I know to avoid conflict with the medical doctors the therapists insist their evaluations are not diagnoses, but I sure can't see the difference). Doctors took advantage of the increasing skill of the physical therapist by delegating much of what had been their work; their prescriptions often just read "provide physical therapy."

The education to be a physical therapist expanded to being a master's degree. Now, in the majority of states if you are in the 80 percent of the adult population with back pain, you can go directly to a physical therapist, get evaluated, and get therapy designed to deal with your problem. I've done it; it works just fine.

The evolution of the profession has not always been smooth. Practicing without a doctor's prescription required a change in the physical therapists' practice act. The medical profession has opposed this change with varying degrees of vigor and success. When we first tried it in Wyoming in 1985, I got the necessary change through the Senate, but a doctor who was a member of the House defeated most of what we wanted and we had to settle for some minor improvements. Physical therapists could measure, test and evaluate, but they could not treat without a physician's prescription.[7] Finally in 2003, the therapists were able to compromise with the Medical Society and get a limited ability to treat without a doctor's prescription.[8]

The physical therapists are typical in another way. As they expanded their scope of practice, they developed a sub-profession, the physical therapy assistant (PTA), which took over many of their old functions, providing many patients with therapy directly and supervising their exercises. The PTA requires a two-year degree and is often trained at a community college. They are naturally paid less than physical therapists and must be supervised by physical therapists.

This kind of subordinate or related profession is very common. As a profession expands, some of its functions requiring less training get delegated to the related profession. The occupational therapists have the Certified Occupational Therapy Assistants (COTAs). The doctors have the physician assistants and the certified nurse practitioners. The ophthalmologists have the optometrists, a related profession that developed independently. The registered nurses (RN) have the licensed practical nurses (LPN) and the certified nurse assistants (CNA). The dentists have the dental hygienists.

The whole process makes considerable sense. The related profession saves the public money because those professionals get paid less because they require less training. By concentrating in particular areas, they often develop technical skills from practice that the lead profession never adequately developed or loses as it goes on to more complicated issues. The result is better and cheaper care for everyone.

Where the subprofession is developed by the lead profession, the process can be quite harmonious. Changes in the practice act often will be required, but they will not be strongly opposed and will pass under the legislative radar screens. When, however, a related profession is pushing into another's turf or seeking to break free from its parent, epic legislative battles can result.

Legislators hate battles over professional scope of practice. They tend to be waged on both sides by professionals who proclaim and deeply believe that their position is right in terms of protecting the public interest. These claims of protecting the public mask the actual concerns of economic interest and professional pride and make it more difficult to reach reasonable compromises.

The health professions are in many ways set up like medieval guilds and react in much the way a guild would when their turf is threatened. Jurisdictional battles between modern labor crafts like plumbers and boilermakers also can be similar. Getting involved in a scope of practice licensure dispute is often a way for a legislator to make one or both sides mad without any offsetting political gain.

Some of the motivation is pure economics. Consider the dispute between the doctors and the physical therapists over practice without referral. Some of the doctors were getting income from seeing patients to provide the referral. This was not a big factor in Wyoming with our physician shortages, but it was a factor. A more important factor was that some of the doctors whose patients needed a lot of physical therapy had hired physical therapists and were making a profit referring patients to their employees. However, the medical opposition to the change went well beyond economics.

Professional pride was clearly involved. The psychology works like this — a person's professional training and licensure go a long way in defining who a person is. It is a status that is gained with considerable work, personal sacrifice and expense. During that training, people are conditioned to believe that their profession is the only one or the best one to provide their services. How could some other person who hasn't made their sacrifices to get their degree of professional knowledge possibly do as good a job? When another profession claims it can do parts of the job perfectly well, the individual self-worth of the original profession is challenged and its members react accordingly. The resulting feelings are often resistant to rational argument and compromise and the politician in the middle gets caught in a no-win political crossfire.

Practice restrictions on who does what often are a source of high health care costs. Unnecessary ones are often a way that special interests run the cost for all of us up without providing real value in return. In Wyoming we hit one in the administration of medications to patients in nursing homes and other institutions. Many of the patients in nursing homes and like institutions are on long-term maintenance medications — blood pressure medication is a common example. These can be given as a routine matter with only rudimentary precautions needed to prevent problems. When the patients are at home, either they or a family member administers the medication. In the institutional setting, individualized packaging and other techniques can be used to prevent mistakes.

In Wyoming our institution for the severely developmentally disabled has a long history of using trained aides to administer medications without problems. In 2003 my committee decided we could reduce costs by eliminating the legal requirement that nurses administer medications in nursing homes and similar institutions. We proposed a bill to allow trained CNAs to do the job. The nurses sprung into violent opposition. We were invading their turf and they didn't like it. In Senate debate, the opposition was led by a widely respected member who is a nurse. She was strongly backed by lobbying from the profession. We were lucky to escape with a law allowing us to continue the practice in the state institution already doing it. We got that much only because the alternative was a significant appropriation to allow that institution to hire more nurses.

In that case, some of the opposition came from the usual professional opposition to having its turf invaded, but a lot of it came from the nature of the nurse's job in the nursing home. There the nurse's job is being defined as administration and filling out government paperwork. The nurses don't like that; most of them went into nursing because they enjoy patient contact. Administering the meds was the device they were using to preserve patient contact. I think if we had a different way of ensuring regular patient contact, we would not have gotten the degree of opposition we had.

We can predict some future licensure battles. Right now the dentists are in the process of creating a shortage of dentists. They have cut back the output of dental schools by about a quarter at a time when the population is aging and growing. Unless there is more technological innovation coming than I think there is, we are headed for a time when people are going to do without needed dental care because there aren't enough dentists to go around. Already much of the Medicaid population is doing without because the dentists have plenty of business without taking the lower Medicaid reimbursements.

I predict in a few years there will be a new sub-profession that will take on some of the uncomplicated tasks like putting in new fillings or replacing old ones that break or fall out. It may develop as an entirely new profession or develop from the current dental hygiene profession, which is starting to seek the ability to practice independent of the dentists. The dental profession will naturally oppose this change, but if more and more people are having difficulty finding a dentist, the dentists will lose this battle.

The psychologists seeking the authority to prescribe medications for their patients will provide another battle. This change is being driven by scientific advances. Many mental illnesses now can be effectively treated with drugs. For many, the combination of drugs and therapy is the most effective treatment. The psychologists are increasingly being trained in the use of drugs so they can understand what the doctors are doing when both are collaboratively treating a patient. This is particularly important when the prescribing doctor is a family practitioner who may not have much training in the use of psychoactive drugs, and this is a common situation. If the psychologists don't get the legal ability to prescribe drugs, they will be cut off from effectively treating their patients and run the risk of being increasingly marginalized.

They already have succeeded in a limited successful experiment in the military and a change in the law in New Mexico and Louisiana. I tried legislation here in Wyoming because we have a problem of too few practitioners in our rural areas, but the psychiatrists rose up in fury, got the rest of the medical profession behind them and beat us. Given our medical shortages, I think the opposition was much more motivated by professional pride than economics. The arguments were couched in terms of protection of the public, but given the successful military experiment, I couldn't see much validity to those arguments. I predict a protracted legislative battle over this proposal.

One word of caution on the licensure issue. There are some market economists who see licensure as pure economic protectionism on the part of the professions. This is going too far. Licensure has a couple of advantages for the public. It does set some minimum levels of competence. If you are away from home and have to see a medical doctor, you can safely assume a certain degree of professional competence. You don't have to do your own investigation of the doctor's skill and training which may be impractical, especially in emergency situations. Second, it gives the professions and the government a device for getting rid of professionals who are grossly incompetent, criminals, or sexual predators. Wyoming recently licensed respiratory therapists.[9] An argument in favor of the legislation I found convincing was that we were at risk of becoming a refuge for criminals and perverts who had been run out of practice elsewhere because we were one of the last states to license that profession.

My summary of all this is that high professional pay is, and will continue to be, an important source of rising health care costs. It is primarily a product of our free labor market rewarding professional education and training. We should not want to change that even if we could. We can and should increase education and training opportunities to ease shortages, but this strategy is slow and expensive. We can and should modify professional licensure laws to remove unnecessary and outmoded restrictions on who can do what. But some of these changes will be made over vigorous opposition from professionals whose monopolies are being invaded. When the legislature gets into a battle over professional licensure, pay attention. Your safety may be at risk but probably isn't. Your wallet, however, almost certainly is. Licensure restrictions are an important cause of our high health care costs.

Chapter 10, Footnotes

(1) Gerard F. Anderson, Uwe E. Reinhardt, Peter S. Hussey, Varduhi Petrosyan, "It's the Prices Stupid: Why the United States is So Different from Other Countries," Health Affairs 22(3): 89-105, 2003.

(2) Joel Hay, Sharon Forrest & Mireille Goetghebeur, "Executive Summary, Hospital Costs in the U.S.," October 15, 2002, report prepared for BlueCross BlueShield Association, page 12. Published by the BlueCross BlueShield Association as part of a book entitled What's Behind the Rise: A Comprehensive Analysis of Healthcare Costs.

(3) Hay et al, Ibid, page 12.

(4) Edward Salsberg, "Making Sense of the System: How States Can Use Health Workforce Policies to Increase Access and Improve Quality of Care," The Reforming States Group, Milbank Memorial Fund, 2003, page 3.

(5) Joanne Lynn, Sick to Death and Not Going to Take It Anymore!, University of California Press and Milbank Memorial Fund, 2004, page 19.

(6) See W.S. 21-19-202(c)(vii) and Chapter 90, Session Laws of Wyoming, 2003.

(7) Session Laws of Wyoming, 1985, Chapter 216.

(8) Session Laws of Wyoming, 2003, Chapter 111. There were various restrictions on the right to treat without a prescription, the most important one being a requirement for a prescription after 12 visits or 30 days, whichever comes first.

(9) Session Laws of Wyoming, 2003, Chapter 168.

Chapter 11

WELLNESS AND PREVENTION

The best way to reduce health care costs is to prevent disease in the first place. This chapter will discuss steps that can be taken to encourage disease prevention.

The good news about prevention is that you don't need the government or any other organization for the most important preventive measures. You can do them yourself. The bad news is you have to do them yourself. You already understand the essentials. Don't smoke. Exercise. Keep your weight reasonable. Avoid illegal drugs and excessive use of alcohol. Use seat belts in cars. These are all things you have to do for yourself; nobody can do them for you.

This chapter will focus on what the government and other organizations can do because the focus of the book is on health policy, but don't let that downplay the importance of what you can do for yourself. Appendix 1 contains helpful suggestions for things you can do yourself, many of which you already know.

The most important thing anyone can do to prevent disease is to stop using tobacco if they either smoke or chew. Tobacco is the major cause of lung cancer and makes almost every other health condition worse, including the Number One killer, heart disease.

Quitting smoking (or using chewing tobacco) is very hard; tobacco is extremely addictive. Years ago I watched my wife quit smoking and that made me very glad I had never started. There are some things that can help, including some drugs and patches, but there is no substitute for an individual quitting and toughing the withdrawal out.

There are some things the government and private organizations can do to help. There are various tobacco cessation programs that can be run by the government or private organizations that do help. Public events like the Great American Smokeouts help. Public and family pressure helps. I know families where the kids make mom or dad smoke outside and that helps. We are gradually making smoking socially unacceptable and that pressure helps.

One of the more effective things the government can do is to raise the tax on tobacco. Even though tobacco is addictive, higher taxes do reduce consumption by adults. It gives some people the extra motivation they need to quit, and for others it reduces their consumption. More importantly it helps teenagers not start. Too many of them don't care about the long-term health consequences, but they do care about having enough money for "music," clothes, cars and attracting the opposite sex. High prices make cigarettes compete with these other priorities and that affects their willingness to start smoking.

The evidence that higher taxes decrease smoking by raising the price of cigarettes is clear. The generally accepted figures come from the federal Centers for Disease Control and Prevention, the CDC: "Economic studies show that a 10 percent increase in the price of cigarettes will reduce overall smoking among adults by about four percent. A consensus view is that for every 10 percent rise in price, there will be a seven percent decrease among young people smoking."[1]

I have pushed two tax increases through the Wyoming Senate.[2] The most recent one raised the cigarette tax to 60 cents a pack. It had the expected effect of decreasing cigarette consumption.[3] I want to go higher.

The chairman of the Senate Appropriations Committee told me when the tax increase was being considered, that if it passed he'd quit just to spite us. It passed and he did, but he has since relapsed. I like John and I'd like to help him. I figure we didn't raise the tax enough to get the job done. Maybe a further increase will provide the necessary extra motivation.

I suppose if we go too fast, we could hurt some low-income individuals, but this is a voluntary tax people can avoid by quitting. If a state goes too high, it can induce too much smuggling from other states, but those are the only restraints that should be recognized.

There are a couple of problems that need to be dealt with nationally. One is Internet sales. They can be used to sell tobacco illegally to children and they can be used to evade state taxes. They are interstate commerce and difficult for the states to stop, tax, or regulate. We will try to deal with this problem at the state level, but we need help from Congress. Another problem is sales on Indian reservations. These can escape state taxes and can therefore be used to evade the taxes. We need to cut deals with the tribes on the subject. If we can get the tribes to levy their own comparable taxes, all will be well. Who gets the tax money is a lot less important than getting the tax levies up.

As the reader can tell, I feel strongly about tobacco. One of my favorite legislative bills was the one my daughter Abby got passed. It happened when she was in fourth grade. She came home from school with a copy of the Weekly Reader, which had an article by Dr. Lewis Sullivan, then Secretary of Health and Human Services (HHS). Dr. Sullivan said the states ought to ban cigarette vending machines because they were a way kids could buy cigarettes. Abby threw the magazine on the dining room table and said, "Daddy, make a law."

I said I would if she would help. I knew I would need help because at that time tobacco sales to children were legal in Wyoming and a bill to make them illegal had been defeated in the House at the previous general session by a vote of 31 to 33.[4]

Abby and I started by meeting with then Gov. Mike Sullivan in his office. In addition to the governor, present were the head of the state public health association and several tobacco lobbyists. The governor and the tobacco lobbyists were willing to support making tobacco sales to children illegal, but opposed the next step of banning the vending machines. Abby was not intimidated by these adults — Wyoming being a small state, she knew most of them; she knew the chief tobacco lobbyist as her friend Jennifer's dad. After the meeting ended, we went upstairs to the Legislative Service Office and had them draft the bill the way we wanted it.

Abby wrote to other fourth graders all over the state and asked them to write their legislators. A significant number of them did. This was very useful, as legislators will think twice about voting against a bill being supported by school kids.

Abby came and testified when the bill was in committee during the session. That was hard, getting up to speak in front of a group of adults in a formal committee meeting, but she did it. We had to compromise by allowing vending machines to remain in bars, liquor stores and mines, all places where children are effectively prohibited. That was a useful lesson in how to compromise an issue without compromising the basics we were seeking. The bill passed overwhelmingly, 25 to 5 in the Senate and 46 to 18 in the House.[5] Very few wanted to stand against the schoolchildren. But I was never able to get Abby to help me on another bill. She knew how to quit when she was ahead. She was the only lobbyist I ever knew who batted 1,000.

One of the best preventive measures a person can take is to get regular exercise. It helps maintain general fitness and health and keep weight down. It can help prevent or ameliorate many problems including heart disease and diabetes. The evidence is that within reason, the more exercise the better. But the evidence also is that even moderate exercise can pay big benefits. This is something people have to do for themselves, but there are some ways the government and the community can be helpful.

For people to regularly get the exercise they need, it must be enjoyable. Walking is good moderate exercise almost everyone can do. My community has developed a long walking path called the Platte River Parkway along the river that runs through town. It goes several parks and even semi-wild areas. In good weather, walking along the parkway is very pleasant and a lot of people do it. It is an example of a community effort that can have both preventive health and simple quality of life benefits for the community.

There are other community and commercial activities that can provide attractive opportunities for people to both exercise and enjoy themselves in the process. Tennis courts, swimming pools, golf courses, and basketball and handball courts all are examples. Water exercise classes in swimming pools can be particularly useful for individuals who have trouble walking long distances due to arthritis or other disability or excessive weight. For bad weather, the shopping malls have taken to encouraging walking. People take advantage of this and reward the malls with more business in the process.

A regulatory thing local governments can do that will help people exercise is insist on sidewalks in new developments. This came home to me a few years ago when I went to a three-day meeting at the National Institutes of Health in the Maryland suburbs of Washington, D.C. I stayed with a family friend who lived about 1-1/2 miles from the NIH campus. I figured I could just walk to the meeting. My hostess insisted that she would transport me. I resisted but she insisted and after the first time I rode with her, I understood why. There were no sidewalks along the route I would have taken. In places, the trees and bushes came right down to the road and the traffic was heavy. Walking was clearly unsafe. The design of the neighborhood prohibited walking and forced the use of cars.

In this same area, however, was an example of a community project like our Platte River Parkway that made walking available and enjoyable. There was an old railroad right-of-way that had been converted to a walking trail. The time I went walking there it was enjoyable and was being used heavily. Of course, parking was a problem for the prospective walkers because the design of the community discouraged their walking from home to the trail.

Obesity prevention is a popular topic among legislators. Recent NCSL meetings have usually included a well attended session on this topic. Getting soft drink vending machines out of schools is a popular proposal at the legislative, school board and community activist levels. The soft drinks are accused (rightly) of being empty calories and healthier substitutes are proposed. A general attack on the use of "junk" foods is often a next step. The problem here is that the label "junk food" is often applied based more on emotion and fashion rather than science. My observation is that many of the so-called junk foods often are harmless or even beneficial when eaten in moderation. Legislative and other regulatory efforts in this area can easily turn into unreasonable intrusions into people's personal freedoms.

Another preventive activity people can do is to get various screenings to catch potential disease problems early so they can be treated before they can cause expensive problems.

One effective practice is the community health fairs that are available in a number of communities. These include a blood draw that leads to a battery of screening tests. The health fair uses its non-profit civic activity status and the volume of business it can deliver to get a cheap price from the labs. The tests can pick up many developing problems, including most commonly thyroid problems, high cholesterol and diabetes.[6] The health fairs can arrange a number of other screenings, including mammograms, PSAs, posture evaluations and hearing tests. They make extensive use of volunteers to keep the costs down. Health fairs are cost effective for most people although they can be abused by hypochondriacs.

For communities without health fairs, developing one would be a good project for civic-minded citizens. In Wyoming they are widely available. Our statewide television station, KTWO, led in the 1980s by its then general manager Bob Price, took a major role in developing ours and continues to promote them. Elsewhere, TV stations and TV personalities often have taken a lead in developing local health fairs.

One thing employers can do to try to hold down health insurance costs is to develop a corporate wellness program. Paying for memberships in a local health club or fitness center to encourage exercise is one popular example. There are various organizations that for a price will run screenings and provide various programs targeted for people for whom the screenings could especially benefit from prevention efforts. My community of Casper has one of these named Be Well. These efforts are more common with larger employers and ones with stable workforces where the employees are likely to remain with the employer long enough for the prevention efforts to impact employer health care costs.

There is some thought that employers can influence the health status of their employees and thus the associated costs by the design of their benefit packages. Dr. Hank Gardner, a benefits consultant based in Cheyenne, has made several presentations to Wyoming legislative committees on this subject. People do respond to incentives and generous disability insurance programs and sick day benefits do induce usage and sometimes medical expenses to justify the usage. Generous benefit designs can encourage the hypochondriacs and malingerers among us. This can be another motivation for the medically unnecessary care problem discussed in Chapter 5.

I suspect the first use of a sick day for a fishing trip probably occurred shortly after the first sick day benefit was provided. This is a problem with human nature that is outside the scope of health policy.

There is another set of screening tests that are potentially quite useful, but are more problematic both because they cost more and because some of them have some risk to the patient. Colonoscopies, scans for aneurysms and other conditions, and cardioid artery scans for stroke risk factors all are in this category.

This book will not attempt to provide a definitive guide to these preventive tests. I do not have the necessary medical expertise, and the field is changing too rapidly as new tests evolve. Instead, this chapter will discuss the principles we should use in evaluating tests and how should we make the useful ones widely available.

The first question is can something be done about a problem if the screening test finds it? The colonoscopy is an example of a test that meets this criteria for being useful. If a cancer is found, there are accepted treatments including surgery and chemotherapy. As with most cancers, the earlier the cancer is found, the more likely the treatment is to be successful. Also, polyps that have the potential to develop into a cancer are removed, preventing them from developing into cancers.

To be useful, a test must look for a problem that is common enough and serious enough and it must find a high enough percentage of the problem to be worthwhile. The screenings for stroke, the carotid ultra sound and the ankle-brachial test, pass this test. The Wall Street Journal quoted Dr. William Finn, chief of vascular surgery at the University of Maryland as saying, "Roughly one-half of all stroke deaths and a lot of the permanent disability could be prevented with the cardioid ultrasound test."[7]

Stroke is a major killer (third behind heart disease and cancer in a conventional listing) and a major cause of disability when survived. Preventing half of the strokes is worth a good deal. This test also meets the first criteria — something practical can be done about results that show a problem. If the cardioid test shows a blockage in the 80 percent to 90 percent range, surgery or cardioid stents are usually required. A 90 percent blockage is a serious condition.

The Wall Street Journal quotes Dr. Kau S. Yadav, director of Vascular Intervention at the Cleveland Clinic, as saying a 90 percent blockage means an annual risk of stroke of more than five percent.[8] Blockages over 50 percent not requiring surgery are typically treated with drugs including aspirin, statins and ACE inhibitors.[9] These also are the treatments that the ankle-brachial tests, sophisticated blood pressure tests that screen for arterial disease generally can lead to. If a person is already on the drugs that could be used, their doctor might advise not to bother with the test on the grounds it would not lead to different treatment.

Another issue to consider about screening tests is the risk that the test itself entails. Some tests are essentially risk free. If elementary sanitary precautions are taken, a test using a blood sample is in this category. The same with an external measurement like a blood pressure test. However, any invasive test will carry some risk and any test involving ionizing radiation carries a risk. Use of the CT scan to screen for aortic aneurysms is an example where the risk from the test could exceed the benefits of the test. Aneurysms are important killers (c. 25,000 deaths per year nationwide), which can be cured by surgery if caught before they rupture. The surgery is not free of risk, but it is much more successful if done before the aneurysm becomes acute; there are specific guidelines about how large the developing aneurysm should be allowed to get before surgery is indicated.

Aortic aneurysms can be detected by CT scans, abdominal ultra sounds, MRIs and echocardiograms. My calculation for CT scans, however, is that in a general screening of the adult population the CT scan would cause between three and four fatal cancers for every fatal aneurysm it found and prevented. However, for someone with symptoms or someone in a special risk category, a doctor might well conclude that a CT scan is worth the risk. I have some family history of aortic aneurysm, looked at the risks, and concluded an abdominal ultrasound (fortunately negative) was the appropriate test for me.

Cost is another issue that must be considered. And the cost is linked to the chance a problem will be found we can do something about and also to the consequences and costs of the problem if nothing is done. For example, there are a number of screenings for very rare problems in newborns that can be done quite cheaply from a blood sample. The diseases can be devastating and very expensive, but can be prevented or

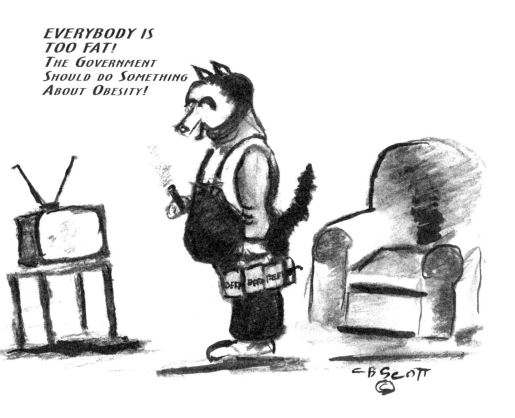

successfully treated if found early. The cost of the test is low, so the cost benefit ratio is good even though the diseases are quite rare. Other tests and scans can be much more expensive. Colonoscopies can cost $1,500 to $2,500. The Wall Street Journal reports the stroke screenings run between $45 and $250 for each test.[10]

If a screening test meets the various criteria — it leads to effective treatment, it's accurate, its benefits outweigh its risks, it's cost effective — what can we do as a matter of public policy to see the test is used by those who can benefit from it?

A popular solution with many legislators will be to mandate coverage of the test by health insurance. This solution was discussed in detail in Chapter 7, Insurance Problems. The problems are that it reaches a relatively small part of the population and the cost to the overall system is higher than other methods due to the excessive insurance administrative costs, especially where the test is relatively cheap.

Another solution I favor is making the most cost-effective tests available to everyone meeting the appropriate criteria (often age or sex). The test would be a "free" public health benefit paid for with general tax revenues. We have used this strategy with many vaccinations with success although we are seeing 70 percent childhood vaccination rates where we want to see 90 percent rates.

Since the state is interested in the general health of the population and the total cost of the health care system, we don't care if the individual tested moves from one health insurance company to another or even if the eventual savings comes to Medicare. Since Medicare pays less than cost, something that reduces the need for Medicare services helps everyone by reducing cost shifting. The opposition to making screening tests "free" public health benefits will be that they will then be paid for with general tax revenues and legislators get blamed if tax rates go up. Some legislators also are opposed to any new government programs on principle.

Another problem with screening tests is that even if they are free to the individual, many people don't get them. People are busy; they don't understand how much good the test may do them. We all procrastinate, and many of us react to the fear the test may find something bad by avoiding the test. It's a bad strategy. What you don't know can very easily kill you, but that's the way we humans are.

Individuals need to keep up on what screening tests may be appropriate for them. You should discuss the issue with your doctor, but beware of three problems. First, has your doctor kept up with the current knowledge on what tests are appropriate? Not all of them do. Second, is your doctor aware of the risks of the test and willing to discuss them? I find many doctors ignore the radiation risks. Those risks are real, even if they are long term and no individual cancer can be traced to a specific radiation exposure. Third, if you come in asking for a test, will the doctor give it to you whether or not it is justified? In this day and age of liability risk, many doctors will take the attitude that the customer is always right on something like a screening test. This could result in spending money on unnecessary tests.

There are many sources of information on what tests are useful. I have found The Wall Street Journal and the popular women's magazines to be the best sources in the news media. With all sources be critical — new tests can be hyped by people who make money from them and fads always are possible.

An effective thing legislatures could do to encourage appropriate screenings is to form a professional committee to study the ones available and recommend to the public which ones they should get. The committee should hold public hearings designed partly to get recommendations from experts and partly to get publicity to the general public and the medical community. The committee should evaluate the screenings on the criteria suggested by this chapter including the risks to the patients, something we too often ignore. It should have a budget for publicizing its findings to both the public and the medical community.

Naturally the committee's recommendations often will be based on the various national recommendations that are available, but having a local evaluation using estimates of the number of local deaths that can be avoided will help persuade people to actually get beneficial screenings. It also may generate the political support needed to deal with the financial obstacles to people getting the useful screenings and help set rational priorities in this area.

This is a brief overview of some of the policy possibilities in the wellness and prevention area. I'm sure there are many creative ideas I have not touched on. This is an area where creativity from individuals, employers and legislators can lead to real improvements in our health.

Chapter 11, Footnotes

(1) Centers for Disease Control (1999), "Decline in Cigarette Consumption Following Implementation of a Comprehensive Tobacco Prevention and Education Program — Oregon, 1996-1998" 48(07): 140-143, February 26, 1999. From http://www.cdc.gov/tobacco/research_data/interventions/mm299fs.htm.

The reader also is referred to F.J. Chaloupka and K.E. Warner, "The Economics of Smoking," NBER Working Paper No. W7047, Cambridge, Mass., 1999, National Bureau of Economic Research, and K.E. Warner, "Health and Economic Implications of a Tobacco-free Society," Journal of the American Medical Association (JAMA), 1987, Vol. 258, No. 15, pages 2080-2086.

(2) Session Laws of Wyoming 2003, Chapter 52.

(3) Marc J. Homer, Zafar Dad Khan and Thomas A. Furgeson, "Impact of the 2003 Cigarette Excise Tax Increase on Consumption and Revenue in the State of Wyoming, Report to the Wyoming Department of Health, Substance Abuse Division," Wyoming Survey and Analysis Center, University of Wyoming, WYSAC Technical Report No. HEG-403, September 2004.

(4) Digest of Senate Journal of the 50th State Legislature of Wyoming, General Session, S. F. 14, page 71. The bill passed the Senate 20-10.

(5) Digest of Senate Journal of the 51st State Legislature of Wyoming, General Session, S.F. 80, pages 118 and 119. The bill became Chapter 76, Session Laws of Wyoming, 1991.

(6) Author's conversation with Sen. John Barrasso, M.D., October 10, 2004. Dr. Barrasso is heavily involved in our local health fairs.

(7) Thomas M. Burton, "Two Simple Tests Can Prevent Stroke, But Few Get Them," The Wall Street Journal, September 24, 2004, page A1.

(8) Burton, Ibid, page A12.

(9) Thomas M. Burton, "Screening for Artery Disease is a Good Idea for People Over 60," The Wall Street Journal, September 24, 2004, page B3.

(10) Burton, "Two Simple Tests . . .," page A12.

Chapter 12

SOLUTIONS THAT DON'T WORK

The goal of health care reform is to produce a system that will provide high quality health care to all Americans. This goal must be achieved at a price our society can afford. I believe that with proper reforms, this goal can be achieved within our current levels of spending. This chapter and the next one will discuss how this can be done. This chapter will identify some popular proposed reforms that will not work and the next chapter will discuss ones that will work.

The caveat that the goal must be achieved at a price we can afford is very important. Our society has other needs and wants and we must strike a reasonable balance among them. As former Colorado Gov. Richard Lamm so eloquently points out, "If public policy allows health care to trump all other considerations, we risk having a medical Taj Mahal amidst massive social squalor. Public policy tries to bring social balance to the total society and cannot allow one category of needs to trump all other social considerations."[1] Lamm's choice of a simile is apt. The Taj Mahal is after all a tomb and it was constructed by a society with massive poverty and squalor.

As a legislator, I find Gov. Lamm's statement rings true. Society does have competing needs. The people of every democratic country have chosen to retain ultimate control of how the balance is struck, including the balance between governmental services and private ones. In the United States, they have delegated the details of the job to a group of elected officials, the Congress, us state legislators, and various local "legislative" bodies like city councils and school boards. The people retain control because they can readily replace us at the next election if we get the balance wrong. This is the essence of the republican form of government that the Constitution guarantees every state.

Because there is a balance we cannot give unlimited resources to any group or purpose, no matter what their ethical or constitutional claims are. If we are to preserve a democratic society where the people have the ultimate control, we legislators cannot yield the decision on where to strike the balance to anyone except other elected officials or the people themselves.

Now, how does this apply to health care? There is a group, including Lamm, that will argue that society must ration health care. In their view the goals of the highest quality health care for all and a health care system society can afford are incompatible. As Lamm says in the conclusion of the paragraph quoted earlier, "No nation or system can meet all the individual needs and desires of an aging, technologically obsessed society by using pooled funds."

The theory is that society cannot afford to give everyone high quality health care — that costs too much. The system must ration care. Currently it rations by denying care to those who can't afford it because they are poor or lack good health insurance. The theory is it would be better if rationing were done on some other "more rational" basis by either private sector bureaucrats (e.g. HMO managers) or government bureaucrats. Presumably the rationing would be based on some kind of a cost per quality year of life saved basis.

The efforts of Oregon under Gov. John Kitzhaber are the most explicit effort we have seen in this area. Oregon went through an elaborate public process to cut some procedures from Medicaid funding in order to get the resources to spread benefits to a larger group of people. The project seems to have fizzled due to public, political and bureaucratic resistance to actually cutting off procedures with significant dollars attached and the pressure from Oregon's budget crisis.

Intellectually, I think the arguments of Lamm and others are hard to dispute, and factually, we in the United States have rationing on the basis of ability to pay. However, as a practical matter, we have no need to ration any needed health care. The key word is needed. Remember we are spending about 50 percent more of our GNP on health care than the rest of the developed world and getting poorer results. In Chapter 3, I discussed the degree of medically unnecessary care in our system. In Chapter 2 on malpractice, Chapter 9 on prescription drugs, and Chapter 10 on workforce issues, I discussed some of the ways various special interest groups are profiting from the system without giving us value in return.

It is my thesis that by cutting back on the medically unneeded care and doing even a halfway job of cutting back on the special interest take, our society can pay for all the medical care all of us need. In this chapter and the next, I will try to separate various system reforms on whether they help with these factors and whether or not they work or cause other problems that make them impractical.

One idea that is periodically tried is price controls or the government setting the prices for health care. The idea is very simple — high prices are a problem so the government will set prices where they are not a problem.

The price control mechanisms already in place turn out to be a major part of the problem with our health care system. Both Medicare and Medicaid set prices below what the services they use cost to provide. The trouble this causes for the rest of the system was discussed in Chapter 6 on cost shifting. The problems that the Medicaid drug price control system causes by holding prices up and interfering with price competition in prescription drugs were discussed in Chapter 9.

Several states have experimented with regulating hospital prices, and Maryland still does. Maryland is unusual also in that the price regulation extends to Medicare charges, something that is legal only if the price regulation is cost neutral for the federal government. What Maryland does is workable only because Medicare reimbursements are high in that state relative to the rest of the country.

If high prices were caused by exorbitant profits being made by hospitals or other institutions with natural monopolies, then price regulation might be useful. If, however, the high prices are due to the high costs imposed by our free labor market, the high costs of R&D and regulatory approval for new drugs and medical technologies, and a litigation risk premium, then price regulations will not produce significant net benefit. The problems lie in the underlying costs and in the degree to which unnecessary services are provided and price regulations do not reach these problems.

In addition to cost shifting, the provider response to government price setting has been two-fold. To keep their income up, they have provided more services. Sometimes they have taken a service they were already providing and split it into different components. This is the process that has led to separate hospital charges for every little thing from providing the rolling stand to hanging IVs to administering aspirin. Accounting for all these unbundled services is one of the engines behind our excessive administrative costs. The other thing they have done is provide more actual service, some of which is medically unnecessary. Both practices run our health care costs up without providing value in return.

One of the most popular reforms that would not work well is the single-payer system. The basic idea is very simple — the government takes over all of health care, manages it and pays for it. The argument is that it has proven to work elsewhere, so why not adopt it here.

I think a single-payer system would be a mistake for two reasons. First, our size and culture have elements that will make it work less well here than elsewhere. Second, it really doesn't work as well elsewhere as proponents suggest.

I concede there are some advantages that come with a single-payer system, especially reducing administrative costs. Our health care administrative costs are twice or more what other countries have.[2] Our complex payment system is the primary cause of this (malpractice defense needs are a secondary cause). It is reasonable to expect that if we did a single-payer system competently, we could cut our administrative costs nearly in half, saving about 10 percent of the total costs or about 1.5 percent of GNP. This is a big dollar advantage to the single-payer system.

Having identified the big savings advantage for the single-payer system, let's now talk about some of the reasons why it would not work well here.

The first reason is our size. Our population is much larger and more culturally diverse than the other countries that use a single-payer system. Roughly speaking, our population is 8-1/2 times that of Canada and 4-1/2 times that of Great Britain. Size makes a big difference because the larger a governmental system is, the harder it is to manage. This is true for private systems, but it is even more true for governmental systems. Our cultural diversity is a further complication because some of our subcultures are sufficiently different that they need different management strategies on a variety of issues. Different management strategies are something a bureaucracy finds hard to accommodate.

A major cause of problems for governmental systems is the management control function. In all large organizations, the work is actually done by subordinate units. The day-to-day decisions required to run the operation have to be made at a local level. The functions of the central administration are to set strategy, allocate resources and develop a system to provide incentives for correct local decision making. The central management then monitors local results to reward good results and correct bad ones.

As size increases there will be more levels of administration. To know which subordinate units are performing well and should be rewarded and which are performing poorly and need corrective action, the central administration needs objective measures of performance. The larger the system, the more important the need is because as size increases, it becomes progressively more difficult for central managers to know personally what the local performance is.

In the private sector, profit is the measure of performance. Subordinate units are judged on the basis of profit or some measure like sales volume or manufacturing cost that relates to profit. The profession of accounting is devoted to the problems of measuring profit and related indicators objectively. As the recent corporate accounting scandals prove, it is possible for people to commit frauds or, I believe more commonly, to use accounting numbers to deceive themselves along with everyone else, but most of the time the system works well.

This system does not work for governmental entities. They generally have no agreed on objective measure of performance. Look at the struggles education is having with the measures required by the No Child Left Behind Act. Some of the opposition to the accountability measures it uses comes from educators who fear their performance is objectively not good enough and will result in personal consequences. The greater source of opposition, however, comes from a valid fear that the measures are not adequate and will measure things the educators cannot control. Tests are likely to measure the incoming abilities and family circumstances of the students more than the performance of educators and the education system.

I argue that this inability to objectively measure performance is the most important reason for the failure of socialist systems like the former Soviet Union. They constructed vast industrial empires that inefficiently produced shoddy goods that were of little value to anyone. They did it not because they were inherently incompetent, but because they could not objectively measure which of the things they did were valuable to their society and which were not.

Our government is not immune to this same problem. My wife, who worked 13 years for the U.S. Public Health Service, says that the government is full of good people, working hard, doing things that don't need to be done.

In health care, the problem is somewhat ameliorated because at the point of service, we have professionals with a clear goal — make the patient in front of them well again. However, health care involves systems that are now complex and are rapidly growing more complex as we learn more about our complex biology. These require management, which requires objective measures that are lacking. Again size makes the problem worse.

This does suggest that if we try a single-payer system, we will do better with one run by the several states like the Canadian provincial system rather than a single national system like Britain has. This federal approach will not eliminate the problems, especially given the size of some of our states, but it will help.

Another cultural problem we have is that at least at the national level, we are in a period of major political corruption. This is not unique in our political experience. We had a similar period between the end of the Civil War and early 1900s. It was during this period that Mark Twain said, ". . . there is no distinctly native American criminal class except Congress."[3] In that period, the politicians were taking personal bribes. With rare exception, that isn't true now. Now they're taking campaign contributions.

Let me explain. For a full-time professional politician, losing an election can have terrible personal consequences. If they lose, they have to find not just a new job, but a new profession. They may in the end be better off, but the transition will be personally trying and most people avoid such things or want to do them at a time of their own choosing when they have the new job or new profession lined up.

Most elections are decided by the group of voters who are relatively apathetic and uninformed, but still care enough to vote. These are the people whom the 30-second TV commercial can sway. Elections therefore often turn on who has the biggest war chest to pay for TV and other advertising. The professional politician wants a big war chest to either scare off competition or win if he gets competition. What has happened at the congressional level is that too many of the professional politicians are for sale to the highest bidder in campaign contributions. They also are very sensitive to special interest groups who might fund or even recruit a challenger.

This has consequences for health care. The AHRQ publishes a practice guideline that says the evidence shows too many back surgeries are being performed. The orthopedic surgeons get offended and contact their representatives in Congress. They are significant contributors to congressional campaigns. The political heat comes on, AHRQ appropriations get threatened, and AHRQ ceases to do practice guidelines because they are too politically controversial. This is a bad enough problem in our current system. Think how much worse it would be if the federal government was the only one deciding which treatments to fund.

We are having a great deal of difficulty dealing with corruption from campaign contributions. Some of the problems are fundamental. How can you objectively tell the difference between the politician who takes a position because he or she believes it is right from the one who takes the position because it brings in campaign contributions? And don't we all have a right to support the election of representatives who agree with our point of view?

We can't abolish the need for campaign contributions because to do so would give incumbents an advantage that no challenger could overcome. People will not, for good reason, vote for an unknown and getting known takes money.

So far the various efforts at campaign finance reform seem to have made the problem worse. Either they were not well thought out or they were too well thought out by those with an interest in the current system. My observation is that the contribution limits have caused the members of Congress to become obsessed with fund raising. They spend too much of their time on it, and turn the actual work of legislating over to staffs, intervening only to insert special interest protections or grandstand on issues the media is hyping.

The problem in state legislatures is less than in Congress, although a few of the full-time professional legislatures may have a problem that approaches that of Congress for the same reasons. With a few exceptions (for example the California Senate), our legislative districts are smaller than congressional districts and we rely more on personal contact in campaigns and less on expensive media.

The majority of legislatures are part time with the members having other jobs providing at least part of their living. They can personally afford to take more chances in elections. The extremes are the citizens' legislatures like Wyoming. Our regular sessions are constitutionally limited to 60 days per biennium with no more than 40 in one year. Our members have to earn their living elsewhere. Most members would be money ahead to lose their next election and stay home tending to business. Our districts are small, so campaigns are cheap. We can tell a special interest to go to hell without serious personal consequences

The whole issue of campaign finance reform is outside the scope of this book.[4] For now we should take it as a given that a single-payer system would be subject to enough special interest legislation to seriously interfere with its ability to do a good job. This kind of a problem is much less important in the parliamentary systems that the rest of the world uses.

Individual members of Parliament personal fates depend on the standing of their party and their standing within the party, not on the size of their personal campaign war chests. Their elections are not as expensive as ours. Parliamentary systems have other disadvantages and I would not want to go to one, but they manage a single-payer health care system better than we would because they are less subject to special interest legislation.

For this reason as well, if we do go to a single-payer system, we should manage it at the state level rather than the national level because the state legislatures are less subject to campaign contribution corruption than the U.S. Congress. If a state yielded too much to special interests and its system was more costly or poorer quality than other states, it would lose businesses and population to those states and the media would have a comparison to point to. A difficulty is the bulk of the financing has to come through the federal government and experience shows the Congress would yield to the temptation to micro-manage and insert special interest protections.

A further problem with a single-payer system is that it would inevitably involve rationing and become immensely unpopular in consequence. The American public did not like it when HMOs tried to ration health care trying to get rid of medically unnecessary expenses. They will like it even less well when government bureaucrats try to ration needed care as well.

The British deal with governmental rationing caused by limited budgets by allowing private health care. The consequence is that they have a class system of medicine with those who can afford it skipping the queue and getting prompt service in the private sector. In Canada, those who can afford it come to the United States to avoid governmental rationing. Our system will refuse nonessential routine care and preventive care to those who can't pay, but will not refuse needed acute care including major procedures. Extensive queues with wealth bypasses would be extremely unpopular here.

The degree of bureaucracy itself would be a major problem for a single-payer system whether it was managed at the national or the state level. Bureaucracies attract people who like to be rigid about following rules and procedures designed for their own convenience, not the customers'. The U.S. Postal Service with its legislated First Class mail monopoly is an example at the national level. It does an adequate job on routine matters, but it can be very insensitive to its customers on anything outside the routine. And for parcels and express mail, at least those of us in rural areas get much better service from its private sector competitors. This problem is not confined to the federal government as anyone who has had to deal with a state department of motor vehicles over licensing issues can attest.[5]

A further difficulty with the single-payer system is the implications it would have for our tax system. Government expenditures for health care now are about 6.9 percent of GNP. Depending on how it was done, especially how much was left for private expenditure, they would rise to between 11 percent and 14 percent of GNP. This would mean a tax increase of at least four percent and more likely five percent or six percent of GNP.

This size of tax increase will have significant effects on our economy. Sure the increase in public expenditures and taxes is offset by a decrease in private health care expenditures, but the money will come from different places and will have different effects on people's incentives. Specifically, higher tax rates decrease people's incentives for economically productive activity. If the government takes too much of what you earn, you are tempted to work less. The wealthy will devote more resources to lawyers and accountants to exploit loopholes in the tax code. Loopholes and tax code quirks will distort our economic incentives so activity and investments are focused in less efficient ways. If the government takes too much of the returns from making capital investments, less will be invested because fewer investments will be adequately profitable. I argue that the higher European taxes needed to pay for health care, and other aspects of the welfare state, are one of the main reasons the economy of the U.S. has so outperformed that of the rest of the developed world for the last two decades.

A further problem with the single-payer system is that the government will set the prices for the health care services it provides. It does this already for Medicare and Medicaid, but the transition to doing it for the whole health care system will be difficult. Now the government tends to pay less than the services cost with the difference shifted to the private sector (see Chapter 6). That will no longer be possible in a single-payer system because there will not be much of a private sector to shift to.

I predict that government bureaucracies will have trouble adjusting to the difference and will destroy a number of our health care institutions in the process. I also predict that government bureaucracies will have trouble compensating the most skilled professionals as well as they now are. The consequence is that some of these skilled professionals will find they can take their services elsewhere in our free labor economy and health care shortages will result. Finally, I predict that government price setting will kill off a significant proportion of the pharmaceutical and medical device R&D, slowing down progress in those areas.

A variation of the national single-payer system has been to do it at the state level. John McDonough, a supporter of single payer, reported on this issue at the 2004 annual meeting of the NCSL and concluded it is not feasible, a conclusion I agree with. It has been tried twice as initiatives in states with that process. In 1994 in California it lost 27 percent to 73 percent and in Oregon in 2002 it lost 21 percent to 79 percent. The main problems are financial. McDonough reports that single payer would more than double the size of state finances. The resulting tax increases would be very unpopular and would make the state uncompetitive with its neighbors.

McDonough also pointed out that with health sector growing at 2-3 times the growth of the economy in general, single-payer costs would grow faster than tax revenues making it a guaranteed source of fiscal instability.[6] McDonough did not point out, but I will, that this same problem applies to a national single-payer system, if tried before health care costs are controlled. McDonough also pointed out that single payer would make the legislature responsible for every problem in health care.

This is trouble because legislatures have difficulty dealing with too many problems at once; building the consensus and coalitions needed to do something effective takes too much time. Look at the difficulty states are having dealing with just the malpractice problem, and we're making more progress than the U.S. Congress is on that issue. Finally, as our experience with HMOs shows, voters will respond negatively to rationing threats whether real or induced by providers afraid of efforts to cut out unneeded care.

My summary is single-payer systems do not generate enough savings from reducing administrative costs and getting preventive care to some who now lack it to offset their other problems. They will likely ration needed care and the resulting political backlash will make it more difficult to deal with the problems of unneeded care. The bureaucratic processes involved are likely to stifle medical innovation. The tax burdens involved are likely to damage the rest of the economy. Our size and political corruption problems mean we will not manage the system as well as the rest of the world does. The single-payer system is not a good solution to our health care problems.

A real disaster scenario is what would happen if the visibly straining private financing of our health care system suddenly collapsed, as it may if the current rate of cost increases continue long enough. Then the national government might decide it had to go to a national single-payer system in a hurry. To do it in a hurry, they would have to expand existing programs. That limits them to two choices — expand Medicare to cover everybody or expand Medicaid to cover everyone not covered by Medicare. If they try to expand the existing Medicare program, its flaws could well become fatal. Because of the tax increases that would be necessary, there would be vast opposition to financing the program adequately.

The current below-cost reimbursement system would cause incalculable financial trouble for health care providers and the regional inequities would set one region of the country against another. Think roughly of the interior of the country against the coastal regions, but the picture is much more complicated than that. In addition, Medicare is much more a fee for service system with all the incentives for unnecessary care that system provides. The resulting mess would do terrible damage to our ability to provide people with decent health care.

If the option of expanding Medicaid were used, the state setting of provider reimbursements would ameliorate the regional disparities that would be a problem with Medicare. However, bringing 50 independent entities on board would take more time and the process would involve a lot of state/federal political conflict. There would be practical problems with states' inability to finance the resulting costs. These would be particularly pronounced in states with constitutional limitations on taxation. Some states might even refuse to participate. It is hard to say which option would be worse, but it is safe to say that, however done, an emergency transition to single payer would be a mess.

Another reform proposal currently popular is the Association Health Plan (AHP). It tends to come from conservatives who are the biggest opponents of single-payer systems. The argument is that if we can free associations from the restrictions of state regulations, they can offer affordable plans to their small group members. As discussed in Chapter 7, there is some validity to this proposal, especially in those states which have gone overboard legislating specific health insurance coverage mandates. However, I point out that most large business is already exempt from the state coverage mandates due to the ERISA law, and large businesses are having serious problems with excessive insurance costs. AHPs and other reforms designed to avoid state regulations are not a silver bullet to solve the problem of too costly health insurance.

I strongly suspect that the mandate that the AHP advocates want to escape is the guaranteed issue provision in the small group reform. If they can avoid this, they can structure their associations to attract healthier groups. They also can get rid of groups that become unhealthy by raising their prices through the ceiling. This is one of the classic ills of unrestrained competition in the health insurance market — insurers competing by avoiding the people who are in the 20 percent of the population with 80 percent of the costs. The consequences will save the healthy groups money.

It also will increase the price of insurance for everybody else and give employers too much of an incentive to get rid of employees with health problems. There was a reason we enacted guaranteed issue in the small group market. If the AHPs succeed in escaping the small group guarantee issue requirements, a lot more people will be uninsurable. State governments will have to pick up the pieces from that problem. To the extent we don't succeed, there will be additional cost shifting from the uninsured driving up everyone's costs.

A further problem with association health plans is that they would escape state financial solvency regulation. As explained in Chapter 7, insurance is subject to special risks from fraud and deliberate or unintentional under pricing. The federal government has not developed the systems that the states have for dealing with this problem. And when a federally exempt insurance organization does go broke, as will happen, the state guarantee funds will not be there to protect the individual insureds. AHPs would inevitably be a personal financial disaster for some of their insureds.

Chapter 12, Footnotes

(1) Richard D. Lamm, <u>The Brave New World of Health Care</u>, Fulcrum Publishing, Golden, Colorado, 2003, page 122.

(2) For a comparison to the Canadian system, see Woolhandler & Himmelstein, "The Deteriorating Administrative Efficiency of the U.S. Health Care System," The New England Journal of Medicine, May 2, 1991.

(3) Mark Twain, <u>Pudd'nhead Wilson, "Pudd'nhead Wilson's Calendar,"</u> (1894), Chapter 8, quoted <u>Bartlett's Familiar Quotations</u>, 13th edition, Little, Brown and Company, 1955, page 678.

(4) For the record, I think we have gone down the wrong path on campaign finance reform with limits. I think we should abolish contributions from anyone other than natural persons and political parties. (i.e. get rid of political action committees, ban corporate and union contributions). A politician can reason with an individual donor in a way you can't with an organization. I think we should abolish the limits on individual contributions. That would make the representatives beholden either to a few individuals with known special or ideological interests or to mass contributions with similar characteristics and free to exercise judgment in other areas. Now they are beholden to a very wide range of special interests.

(5) In Wyoming, we have partly solved this problem by delegating the vehicle licensing function to local elected officials who we can replace if they make it too much of a hassle.

(6) John E. McDonough, DPH, former Massachusetts legislator now with "Health Care for All" an advocacy group. Presentation entitled "Can States Make Universal Health Care Happen? No, but Don't Let That Stop You," NCSL annual meeting, July 2004.

Chapter 13

SOLUTIONS THAT DO WORK

The theme of this book is that there is no single solution, no magic silver bullet that will solve all the problems with our health care system. There are many steps, however, that if taken together can improve the quality of our health care and bring the cost of the system and its rate of cost increases down to something our society can live with. The discussion of many of the steps that need to be taken is embedded in the earlier chapters. This chapter will briefly recap them and discuss some of the major reform proposals that have promise.

The previous chapter discussed the goal of health care reform — a system which provides all Americans with the care they medically need at a price our society can afford — as a preface to discussing several proposals that will not work.

A key to the success of reform proposals is how well they align the incentives in the health care system with the ultimate objective — producing high quality health care. A second key is how well they make high quality care something everyone can afford.

Health Savings Accounts (HSAs) are a reform our country is going to try because Congress passed the necessary legislation. It was part of the Medicare Prescription Drug Improvement and Modernization Act of 2003[1] and the new tax advantaged account became available January 1, 2004. The accounts are tax-free for employers, and for employees depositing funds, their earnings are tax-free, and their use for health care is tax-free. The National Conference of State Legislatures (NCSL) reports that supporters view HSAs as a way for consumers to pay for routine health care costs before a standard high deductible insurance policy kicks in. The Health Savings Account is an update on the Medical Savings Account (MSA), which Congress passed as a pilot program in 1996. Many of the states can be expected to follow suit. Twenty-six states had MSA legislation and as of July 2004, four have passed HSA legislation.[2]

The HSA can be seen as a part of the push for "consumer driven" health care because it is a device to encourage consumers to pay directly for their medical expenses. Chapter 8, Competition in Health Care, discussed the strengths and weaknesses of consumer driven health care.

The HSA also can be seen as a response to the trend of employers increasing employee premiums, co-pays and deductibles due to rising health insurance costs. Without the HSA, these are paid with after tax dollars and amount to a hidden tax increase for employees.

The problem with the HSA is that health care costs are so concentrated in a relatively small percentage of the population. We discussed earlier the figures that 30 percent of the population accounted for 90 percent of the costs and 70 percent had 10 percent of the costs.[3] At the 2004 NCSL annual meeting, Scott Leitz of the Minnesota Department of Health reported that 50 percent of the population incurs only three percent of the total costs. We can expect the high cost part of the population will either avoid the HSAs entirely or use them up and rapidly reach their traditionally insured third-party payer benefits.

For these reasons, the comments by Halvorson and Isham that MSAs are not exactly a silver bullet because they have the potential of saving only about one percent of the total costs (10 percent of the 10 percent of costs incurred by 70 percent of the population) apply to HSAs as well.[4] They even could cost some businesses more in the short run as too many employees who now have no or very small medical costs can collect more in employer HSA contributions than they cost in direct medical costs.

Another problem with the HSAs is that Congress and the IRS bureaucracy have put in place enough restrictions and regulations to reduce or eliminate their value for some people. How large this problem is, is not set clear.

At the 2004 NSCL annual meeting, John McDonough denounced HSAs as "snake oil." He called them a device to get employees to accept high deductibles. He reported that the tax savings involved are relatively small for most people. His figures show an annual tax savings of only $300 for a family with an adjusted gross income of $50,000 (15 percent of $2,000) with the savings rising to $615 for an adjusted gross income of \$150,000.[5] These figures are a byproduct of the fact that the tax cuts of recent years have made the income tax very progressive with the tax burdens concentrated in the wealthy part of the population.

By including HSAs in the "Solutions that Work" chapter, I obviously disagree with McDonough. The high deductibles were going to happen anyhow as employers respond to rising health insurance costs, so softening the impact on employees is a good thing. I think the estimate that HSAs will save one percent of total costs by making consumers more cost conscious is probably in the right ballpark. The savings could be more if consumers can save more than 10 percent or there are some savings in the 30 percent of the population with 90 percent of the costs. Even if the savings are as high as three percent or even four percent, the claim that this is no silver bullet still holds.

I think there may be two other positive effects. The HSAs should lead to many small health care bills being paid directly rather than turned into insurance claims. In the nature of paper shuffling, many of the administrative costs are more on a per claim than a size of claim basis. Having patients paying small bills directly should reduce the administrative costs for both the providers and insurance companies, an important factor for a system with the excessive administrative costs ours has. These savings could be lost if the system encourages individuals and providers to submit all small bills to insurers anyway just to prove deductibles are being met. The second savings are more speculative. A significant part of the population will have positive balances in their HSAs. Will this make them more likely to get preventive care that will reduce later risks?

An additional reform could enhance the savings from HSAs by enabling them to be used for larger expenses. It would allow HSAs to be used to buy health care "on time" like we buy so many consumer goods. The HSA could be used for a much higher limit of expenses with the deficit financed by a loan. There would then be a payroll deduction to pay off the loan. The deduction would be limited to a percentage of gross pay, which most people could afford. It should be made tax deductible.

There could be some employer sharing of a percentage of the risk involved. The laws would have to be modified so the deficit followed the employee from one job to another the way deductions for child support are supposed to. This could make employees cost conscious about health care costs over a larger range of expenditures, but I still think a majority of expenditures would be outside the reach of the HSA and covered by third-party payers.

In summary, HSAs and other potential "consumer driven" plans, while useful, are only a small part of the answer to our health care cost problems.

Another solution for many people is a well run HMO. HMOs are in disrepute due to the excesses that came with the rapid HMO expansion in the 1990s, but they continue to have the potential of being a high quality, cost effective solution to the problems of our health care system.

The modern HMO got its start in World War II when Henry Kaiser put together an organization to provide health care for the employees in his defense industries. He needed an incentive to attract skilled workers and could not do it with more pay due to wartime wage and price controls. Kaiser's original HMO evolved into what is now known as a staff model HMO.

That HMO model owns most of its own hospitals and clinics, and most of the doctors it uses are its own salaried employees. It is paid a fee per month per enrollee regardless of whether the enrollee uses services or not, the so-called "capitated payment." The organization thus has an incentive to maximize preventive care to avoid expensive problems.

An updated literature synthesis published in Health Affairs found that people in group/staff model HMOs were more likely than those in non-managed care plans to obtain preventive services, but this was not true for the non-staff model HMO.[6]

All HMOs have an incentive to avoid unnecessary care because it costs the organization money rather than earning more as it does in fee for service. The staff model HMO has an advantage in this respect because to the extent it is staff model; it is not contracting with an outside organization that may have the fee for service incentive to provide unnecessary care. In addition as a large organization, it can insulate its individual provider employees from the worst excesses of the tort liability system and thus avoid part of this incentive to provide unnecessary care. I say part because the organization itself has an incentive for defensive medicine.

It also has an incentive to run effective error reduction and quality control programs to avoid the extra care associated with errors. This is largely independent of the malpractice system, because the bringing of a malpractice case has so little to do with the presence or absence of an actual medical error.

With competent management, the staff model HMO can integrate a patient's care, mandating and enforcing teamwork among relevant professionals and getting rid of professionals unwilling or too arrogant to function as part of a team. It can install, and most effective HMOs have installed, an electronic patient records system to facilitate these goals. These are major advantages for a well run HMO.

In its 2004 survey of health care finance, The Economist reports that Richard Feachem, now executive director of the Geneva-based Global Fund to Fight AIDS, Tuberculosis and Malaria, led a study which compared Kaiser in California with the British National Health Service. The study found Kaiser achieved better performance with roughly the same level of resources per person.[7] Since Britain spends less than half as much on health care as the U.S. does[8] and gets better overall results, this comparison suggests Kaiser has a major advantage in both cost and quality over the rest of the U.S. health care system.

Feachem is reported as attributing the Kaiser superiority to better integration of the elements of the health care system, something a staff model HMO is certainly in an organizational position to do. He is quoted as saying, "There is no perfect system in the world; every one has serious flaws and makes serious mistakes which people suffer from, but Kaiser comes closer to an ideal than any system I know."[9]

As discussed in the earlier chapter on competition, HMOs got in trouble due to their contracting problems with providers and their incentives to cut corners, deny needed care and avoid high cost patients. The staff model HMO avoids most contracting problems by using more "in house" providers and facilities, but they are likely to have to contract for some services. They do have the same incentives to deny care and avoid high cost patients as any other HMO. These have to be dealt with by a combination of competent and ethical management, marketplace rewards for good performance and government regulation.

During the rapid expansion of HMOs, different models arose which had few or no owned facilities and employed providers, and which relied heavily on contracting with existing facilities and independent providers. These had a market advantage of offering the consumer a wider choice of providers, but they lost much of the opportunity to integrate services and imported some of the worst fee for service incentives. They also often were managed by people with insurance backgrounds who did not abandon some of the worst habits of insurance companies.

There is a significant number of people in well managed HMOs. Kaiser Permanente alone has 8.2 million Americans enrolled, and there are other HMOs with similar quality. However, there are other HMOs that do not perform as well as the best ones. In addition, HMOs do not appear to generally be successful in rural areas with smaller markets. There once was an apparently successful one based in rural North Dakota (Hettinger), but it did not survive an aberration in Medicare reimbursement. The problem was eventually fixed, but the HMO did not have the size to wait out the problem.

I personally enrolled in an HMO in 1969 when I went to work in Washington, D.C. I was with it five years and was satisfied with its performance. I believed it was a reasonable way to ensure a minimum quality of care in a strange community where I did not have the personal contacts to ensure finding a good quality physician in the fee for service community.

I think that eventually the better HMOs may beat out the poorer ones in the competitive marketplace. A key to reaching this outcome is developing better information on the quality of the care the HMOs provide. There are various efforts to give the consumer (and the employer purchaser) information on quality of outcomes produced by competing organizations. These include the Health Plan Employer Data and Information Set (HEDIS) data set, various state reporting requirements, the efforts of the Leapfrog group and other employer groups.

HEDIS is one of the more important quality measurements. It was developed by the National Committee for Quality Assurance (NCQA). Cutler, a Harvard economics professor, reports NCQA started as an effort by managed care insurers to fend off federal quality monitoring and originally had the goal of deterring inquiries into true quality. He reports that in the early '90s NCQA had a change of heart and started to measure quality of medical care for real. He says insurers care about the HEDIS ranking, advertising positive results and taking corrective action to deal with negative ones. He reports HEDIS has improved use of beta blockers after heart attacks, diabetes treatment, breast cancer treatment and cholesterol screening.[10]

Cutler makes paying for quality the cornerstone of his reform proposals. He reasons that you get what you pay for and we will get better quality if that's what we pay for. His chapter on "Paying for Health" contains a very good description of the efforts to measure quality, their problems and the problems of keeping providers from manipulating the data, which they will try if that's how they are paid.[11]

I differ with Cutler in two respects. I think he underestimates the difficulty of measuring quality. His discussion of the problems of measuring quality is right on target but he assumes, as economists are wont to do, that these problems will be easier to solve than they will be. Also, there is the problem of the cost of the measurements. Cutler says, ". . . plans that require measuring quality inherently involve increased administrative expenses. I am not particularly concerned by this, however. Fundamentally the goal is to get medical care to the right people. If that involves an increased administrative burden, that is an appropriate cost." [12]

Our system already has a major problem with excessive administrative costs. To some extent the value of measuring quality makes the additional administrative cost involved worth the cost. But we do need to be deeply concerned about the size of the administrative cost increase needed to measure quality with the precision that Cutler's proposals need.

If, however, our goal is not to pay on the basis of quality, but to identify the organizations whose corporate or medical culture results in high quality care, we can use much less perfect measures of quality that are cheaper to produce. We still need to take steps to prevent data manipulation and deal with risk adjustment. We just don't need the degree of precision that a payment formula would require. We can live with the kind of gradual improvement in quality measures that the real world is likely to produce.

For those of us hoping for a free market solution to our health care system problems, increasing the availability of good data on quality and increasing its use in deciding among competing providers is key.

The efforts to improve quality data and getting the majority of HMOs to replicate the features that make the best ones work both require time. The Economist quotes Francis Jay Crosson, who heads the physicians' side of Kaiser Permanente, as saying that the company's culture developed over many years and could not be replicated elsewhere overnight just because insurers required it.[13] I would add that the systems and organization structure that many HMOs adopted are sufficiently different from the Kaiser structure that they should not be expected to replicate the Kaiser results no matter how much time is used.

For individuals (and employers) who have access to a well managed HMO, that appears to be a successful answer to our health care problems. The problem is identifying the well-managed HMO. From the evidence I have seen, I think a well managed HMO is likely to be a staff model, but not all staff model HMOs are well managed and I suspect not all well managed HMOs are staff model ones.

The marketplace may eventually sort out the best HMOs from the bad ones. As discussed above, objective performance data will be very important in this process. As this happens we can expect the best HMOs, the ones that really enhance value, to grow and the bad ones to decline. The worst ones may even eventually wind up in the hands of the formal undertaker of the capitalist system, the bankruptcy courts. Whether this happens or not depends in good part on whether employers and the government look beyond price to quality of services.

This in turn partly depends on employees, their unions, and voters and legislators putting pressure on for measurable quality. As one who deals with the government, I suspect the private sector will be more effective in this than the government. It appears the process will take significant time. It will not help many of us in rural areas where there is no access to HMOs. Thus, the well managed HMO, while helpful to many, cannot be the complete answer to our health care problems.

As discussed in Chapter 2, malpractice reform is one of the keys to our total health care reform. The Medical Errors Commission reform proposed in Chapter 2 has the potential of eliminating the defensive medicine cause of our medically unnecessary care and greatly reducing medical error. I would put it at the top of any list of health care reforms.

Defensive medicine caused by the tort liability system is only one of the causes of unnecessary medical care. The fact that providers and the sellers of medical technology make money from unnecessary care is another cause. Health insurers will periodically try to stop the worst of the excesses. The Wall Street Journal reported on an effort by the western Pennsylvania Blue Cross Blue Shield provider to improve quality and eliminate unnecessary scans (MRI, CT, PET). It reported the insurer figured it could save 20-25 percent a year in imaging costs by reducing misread and unnecessary tests. The article reported on the provider opposition that was developing. It also reported that in 2003, plans with imaging controls averaged 69 CTs per 1,000 people while those without controls averaged 115 CTs per 1,000. The MRI difference was similar but smaller (58 vs. 76). [14]

There is clearly significant money at stake in this effort as well as patient safety. The extra CT scans done in plans without controls will cause between two and three fatal cancers for every 100,000 patients enrolled in 2003. These cancers will occur over the lifetime of the patient, not in the year the exposure took place. At the same time, if the controls are eliminating needed scans, patient safety can be compromised that way. My guess is that the effort to control scans will bring providers and possibly even patients complaining to legislators and, if the law permits, suing in the courts. What should we do about it?

I have two suggestions. The easiest and cheapest is to get ready access to the scientific evidence on what is needed and what is not by arranging universal access in your state to the databases of the Cochrane Collaboration. Through our state library, Wyoming has done this. Getting it is simple and cheap; training people to use the databases to find what they need to know is more difficult. A second suggestion is to have each state create a small operations research group to study issues like this.

In conjunction with a medical peer review panel, a group of this nature could be assigned to review issues as they arose. They could examine practice patterns, identify the common circumstances in which scans were used, review the scientific evidence on when they were needed and when they were not, and then come up with a guideline for what is appropriate and what is not. Referring issues to a group like this would be a more productive approach than getting the legislature or the courts into the practice of medicine through a coverage mandate or a lawsuit with the result that the law sets forth what the medical practice should be. Referring issues to such a review organization would allow legislators to do something effective for upset constituents without making a law that could have unfortunate consequences. There should be additional ways to encourage evidence-based medicine to reduce unnecessary and ineffective care.

A third area where unnecessary care can be reduced is end of life care. This is an area where hard and fast rules are difficult because individual circumstances vary. Some cases should be fought with all the weapons in the medical arsenal because real success is possible. In others, aggressive medical intervention will amount to high tech torture and the patient will still die without gaining additional quality life. The best thing the government can do in these circumstances is stay out of the way. The decision making should be left to the patients, their families and their health care providers. This is no place for either the courts or petty bureaucrats. We should allow the patients to set advance directives and see that their wishes are followed.

Institutions like Hospice that provide supportive and palliative care to those with terminal illnesses should be encouraged. I think if we can do a better job of educating people on what the realistic options are, they will do a better job of reducing unnecessary care and improving the quality of the remaining life for those with terminal illnesses. This is something all of us — health care provider, government official and informed citizen alike — can contribute to.

Market based reforms of prescription drug purchasing as discussed in Chapter 9 are another key set of improvements. Where a third-party payer is involved, these include well done preferred drug lists or formularies. Where the individual is involved, programs like Wyoming's PharmAssist, which use pharmacists to give the individual the necessary information to make the market work, are needed. The rewards from an effectively functioning market in prescription drugs make it well worth having the government spend a little money getting effective information to the consumer. Combined with a program like this, the prescription drug area is one where consumer driven health care has the greatest chance of making a significant improvement.

Finally, something needs to be done to provide health insurance coverage for the uninsured. They get inferior health care because they are uninsured and can't afford the preventive care and the care for minor problems that the rest of us get. When the minor problems, like untreated high blood pressure, grow into major problems that lead to preventable hospitalizations, the rest of us are stuck with the cost via the cost shifting phenomenon (see Chapter 6).

The reader is warned, however, to be wary of claims that all the poorer health outcomes among the uninsured are because they are uninsured. There is a good case that to the extent the uninsured are uninsured because they are poor, they also are less intelligent and this causes poorer outcomes. In our society, IQ and wealth are correlated. Lower IQ also translates into poorer ability to follow doctors' orders, manage chronic diseases and avoid risky behavior like smoking and sedentary lifestyles.[15]

Being uninsured is a source of financial worry for many people and is a leading cause of personal bankruptcy. The whole mess is a disgrace for a country as rich as ours.

A word of caution about the data on the uninsured. Most estimates of uninsured are based on the estimates generated by the Census Bureau. The Census includes people eligible for Medicaid and the State Child Health Insurance programs (SCHIP) but not actually enrolled as uninsured. This significantly exaggerates the size of the uninsured problem because these people could get coverage if they get sick and need it. These government programs are different from private insurance — they have no pre-existing condition periods; you can get sick and then get enroll and still be covered. Devon Herrick of the National Center for Policy Analysis has estimated that as many as 14 million of the uninsured are in this situation.[16] This would be 31 percent of the 45 million uninsured the Census Bureau estimated as uninsured for at least part of 2003.

Who are the uninsured? They are not the elderly. The elderly are covered by Medicare. That coverage has some holes and there are people who can't afford the Medicare supplemental policies and don't get the Part B coverage, but the basic Medicare coverage provides health coverage for the elderly.

Relatively few of the uninsured are children. Between the Medicaid program for the poor and the Child Health Insurance Program (CHIP) for the not quite so poor, most of the children whose parents can't afford insurance can get coverage if they are sick and need it. The safety net isn't perfect. The eligible income level for CHIP varies from state to state and there are some children whose parents have too much income for CHIP and don't have insurance through work or can't afford what's offered.

All children where family income is any question have access to preventive vaccination through the public health system. Various screenings, especially for problems related to educational ability like vision and hearing problems, are provided by the public schools. Under the federal Individuals with Disabilities Education Act (IDEA), any children with developmental problems that impair their ability to get an education get a wide array of free services (such as needed speech therapy, physical therapy, occupational therapy to mention a few) through the school system. This is a federally mandated program, but state and local special education budgets provide most of the funding.

Many of the people with the worst chronic illnesses are already covered by government programs and are therefore not included in the uninsured. People who have worked the necessary minimum to be eligible for Social Security (10 years) and who have disabling problems that prevent them from working further get Medicare coverage. There are periodic disputes over individual eligibility and the process of getting on the programs is slow and sometimes difficult, but the coverage is there and is widely used. Someone who is disabled by the progression of a disease like MS is a typical example of a person getting health coverage via this mechanism. People who are afflicted with AIDS have a special set of government programs aimed at that disease.

Formerly many people who had a pre-existing medical condition could not get health insurance and were uninsured. This problem, while not eliminated, as been greatly reduced by government reforms. Many states, including Wyoming, have created subsidized uninsurable pools for these individuals. The problem with these is that their premiums are high (anywhere from 125 percent to 200 percent of the ordinary market premium), but they do enable individuals to get coverage. A second, more important, reform has been the guarantee issue requirement in the small group market (firms with 2-50 employees). This reform prevents insurers from refusing groups with a high risk individual or forcing that individual out of the group.

The uninsured are typically working age adults in households where someone is employed. The 2003 Census data show almost 15 million (33 percent of the total) in households with more than $50,000 in income and 18.8 million (42 percent) between the ages of 18 and 34.[17] There is some overlap in these categories as combined with the Medicaid and SCHIP eligibles, and they add to more uninsured than the Census Bureau found.

Many of the younger uninsured believe (rightly) that their risk of serious medical problems is low. Most of them will be in the 50 percent of the population that incurs three percent of the health care costs. At their ages they need little routine or preventive care and can pay for what little then need. They haven't yet acquired many assets they would lose if they lost the gamble and were forced to bankruptcy by medical bills. They take a calculated gamble that they can do without health insurance and the rest of us will pick up the tab (via hospital cost shifting) if they lose.

The uninsured also include some individuals who are temporarily unemployed between jobs and who either could not afford the continuing coverage from their former employer (COBRA) or took a calculated risk to do without health insurance while they searched for a new job.

The uninsured who are the biggest problem are adults between 40 and 65. Because of age, they are at higher risk for serious illnesses and may need and not get preventive care that could prevent serious problems. They include many who are self-employed or run very small and start-up businesses. These people often cannot afford insurance and may be in the individual market where pre-existing conditions can prevent them from buying insurance.

The fact that most of the uninsured are either able bodied working age adults, usually employed, or in families with one or more members with this characteristic is a key to the design of a program to covered the uninsured. It can be tied to the workplace and to employment.

A second factor governing the design is that insuring the uninsured will cost so much that no entity can afford the whole cost. This includes the federal government, unless it is willing to impose a significant tax increase.

A third is that John McDonough is right, the cost of health care is rising so fast, and historically has done so, that a program to insure the uninsured is likely to be a source of financial instability. He was speaking of state governments, but his analysis applies to the federal government and potential private sources as well. My conclusion is that this means any serious long-term effort to insure the uninsured must be accompanied, preferably preceded, by serious efforts to restrain the growth in health care costs.

My recommendation is that insuring the uninsured should be done as a four-way partnership between the federal government, the state governments, employers and uninsured individuals with each bearing a share of the costs. There are two reasons for doing it as a four-way partnership. One is simply by splitting the cost four ways; we have a better chance that all can afford it. The second is that by having four payers, we have four sources of cost control ideas and four sources of political pressure to control costs.

The states should take the lead in structuring the actual programs as the units of government most responsive to the public will and sensitive to local problems. The federal government is too hampered by its size, the degree of partisan gridlock in Washington, and the degree of corruption in the Congress of the United States. Private entities can't do it because laws are required.

I envision using the Medicaid program as the basis for the reform. It already has a federal/state cost sharing mechanism that varies with the wealth of the states. The federal government pays at least 50 percent of the costs and then may pay a share above 50 percent depending on a complicated formula that varies depending on the wealth of the state and its ability to pay. The formula isn't perfect, but it has been in place for nearly 40 years and I have heard surprisingly little complaint about its relative fairness to the several states.

Certainly in my state of Wyoming it has done a reasonable job of increasing the state share when we are doing well and increasing the federal share when we are doing poorly. The changes in our federal/state share do tend to lag the changes in or actual economy, which I suppose is inevitable. The program also has a long history of accommodating a significant degree of state innovation and experimentation while retaining federal oversight of the basics which is a useful pattern.

For the poorest segment of the population, I would leave the program largely as it is now. I would change the law to allow the states to simplify eligibility to make all individuals eligible on the basis of poverty instead of the current categorical system, which allows some individuals to fall through the safety net. I also would allow for somewhat higher deductibles or co-payments even for this poorest group to deter some usage excesses (like inappropriate emergency room usage) and to encourage use of generic drugs. These reforms will depend on the U.S. Congress passing a law, but fortunately they are not critical to the success of the program.

For the working poor segment of the population, I would expand Medicaid eligibility. Exactly how far to go could be left to state discretion. I suggest something at or slightly below the statewide average wage, something between 200 and 300 percent of the federal poverty level. The expansion of Medicaid eligibility is done through a Medicaid state plan amendment and is the kind of plan amendment the federal government routinely approves. The states historically have set Medicaid eligibility levels when they go above the federal minimums as many have. The people eligible in this enhanced category should be required to work as a condition of eligibility. This is consistent with the philosophy of our successful welfare reform and is necessary to make the financing work. Recall that the disabled and chronically ill who are unable to work for medical reasons are already taken care of by other government programs.

The work requirement can be done with a Medicaid waiver if the administration in Washington is willing to approve. Medicaid waivers require that the states show cost neutrality. This one will save money if compared to what the expanded program would otherwise cost although the total package of the waiver and the plan expansion will cost more. Whether or not it is allowed is a matter of HHS interpretation and does not depend on the Congress changing the law. To get the uninsured as partners I would recommend either enhanced deductibles and co-payments or a sliding scale employee contribution or both.

The purpose of this is to make the Medicaid insurance more like private insurance and to avoid the financial penalty for employees improving their wages that will occur if exceeding the threshold for Medicaid participation results in a big loss of benefits. I expect most of this can be achieved through the waiver process and will not require congressional action. To deal with the problem of young people avoiding coverage, a small tax could be put on wages, possibly equal to their sliding scale Medicaid premium, if they did not have health insurance. This is justified because otherwise the rest of us get stuck with the cost of their major medical problems if they lose their no health insurance gamble.

The additional state costs of the system could be financed in whole or in part with an employer tax that would take the form of a pay or play mandate. The tax would be calculated either as a percentage of payroll or per employee. The aggregate costs of providing employee health coverage would be deducted from the total tax due for all covered employees, a tax credit system. Depending on state financial circumstances, the tax level for low wage workers would be close to or less than the average state share of the Medicaid expenditures for those employees. This should be significantly less than the employer's cost of providing them health insurance.

The employer should pay no tax for any employee with decent coverage because the cost of the coverage should exceed the size of the tax and the cost of coverage would be directly deducted from the tax owed. There will be some tax collected due to high wage workers who refuse coverage because they are on a spouse's policy. I expect that fairly rapidly employers will work out cost sharing arrangements to put a stop to this problem.

Employers would be encouraged to enroll low wage employees in the Medicaid program. The result would be a savings for those employers who had been providing decent health coverage and an additional expense for those who had not. The tax would be a general tax covering all employers, including those whose health plans are ERISA-exempt. There could be legal trouble over the ERISA exemption especially if the states tried to use the deduction method to regulate the contents of plans otherwise ERISA-exempt from state regulation. I think the states would prevail unless they tried something unreasonable in the deduction area for the ERISA-exempt employees. If I am wrong and the system could not cover ERISA-exempt employers, then the Congress would have to modify that law for reform to work.

If a tax is used to pay for the expanded Medicaid program, it should be set annually or biennially in the state budget bill at the same time the Medicaid budget is set. This would make it easier to adjust as costs rose and bring political pressure to control Medicaid costs. Business would have an incentive to help control Medicaid costs because these would have a direct impact on their tax rates. The political clout they would bring to the legislative process would help counter political pressure from providers and lawyers opposed to the reforms necessary to control costs.

A private sector council with both business and labor representatives should be created to work on both cost and quality issues in the expanded Medicaid program. The states could experiment with what powers this council should have to enhance quality and control costs and how it could tie in with private sector insurance issues.

Use of an explicit employment tax will cause political difficulties for this program in many states. A few states, including Wyoming, might be able to do it without an additional tax.

However, since the tax will save money for those employers with low wage employees who are currently on good health plans, the opposition to it should be divided and it should be supported by parts of the business community. This is the advantage of using the Medicaid program with its federal cost share to finance the low wage workers; the state needs only to fund the state share through taxes. This is also a reason for insisting recipients work — the state needs the tax revenue to finance the state share. We already have the non-working very poor on the Medicaid program; if we get a new non-working group on Medicaid, there could be a big hit on state budgets.

COBRA coverage is now often too expensive when someone loses their job and the resulting coverage suffers from adverse selection problems. Those who really need it pay the costs and those who think they can stay healthy long enough to find another job with insurance don't bother. In the new system it would be relatively easy to extend the Medicaid coverage through the period covered by unemployment insurance for those on Medicaid and otherwise subject to a work requirement. For the higher wage workers, the states could do something to subsidize their COBRA coverage for a limited period of unemployment.

The system I am proposing is relatively close to what Maine is trying as its Dirigo Health Plan. Maine's experience is likely to be instructive in how far the states can go toward this system under existing federal law with an unwilling federal Medicaid program. Dirigo Health's financing is a potential problem. For local political reasons, Maine was unwilling to use a tax to finance it and is depending in good part on savings from reducing the numbers of uninsured. I will be surprised if these savings are large enough or easy enough to capture to finance the program.

This new system I am proposing would not quite be universal coverage, but it would be very close to it. With the expanded Medicaid program, it would bring in most people who cannot now afford health insurance; the pay or play mandate would deal with the employers who do not now offer insurance. A few people would remain outside the system — able-bodied, working age adults who refuse to work enough to qualify and a few higher wage employees, mostly younger ones who are willing to gamble they will not get sick. There will be a few higher wage people with employers who would rather pay the tax than incur the extra cost of offering health insurance. These employers will face potential labor market problems and most will offer enough either through HSAs or very high deductible policies to provide coverage whose costs reach the level of tax imposed.

This proposal has the advantage that it can adapt to both the presence and absence of managed care and HMOs in the market. The current Medicaid program frequently uses managed care where it is available, but it also works for those of us with no managed care. The proposal is compatible with the use of HSAs for employees remaining with private insurance coverage and could be made compatible with the use of HSA accounts or something like them for those on Medicaid, if experience proves HSAs provide enough savings to justify the effort.

As was discussed earlier, no state by itself can achieve universal coverage. This proposal with its four-way financing, is feasible, provided the cost increases can be brought under control. It is important to have the private financing, the tax imposed on business not providing insurance, closely tied to the cost of the Medicaid program. This will bring political pressure to control costs that will offset the pressure from provider groups opposed to controlling costs.

Implementing this program requires state legislation. That in turn requires public support and support from that part of the business community which will save money. It needs support from the administration in Washington to get the necessary state plan amendments and waivers approved, although it is possible that enough could be forced through the courts given the current Medicaid law. There are some things the Congress could do to help, but fortunately it appears congressional action is unnecessary. This is very important given the extent Congress is currently dysfunctional.

This proposal can be implemented one state at a time. In doing this, there is the threat that some businesses will move to other states to avoid the employment tax involved. Opponents will threaten this, but if the reform is enacted, little of the threat will be carried out. Since the tax will save money for businesses with a good employee health plan by being cheaper than the cost of the health plan, the business that are the foundation of most states' economy will not want to move. Most of the ones paying more will be retail firms, small service firms where moving is not an option, and small start-ups.

The benefits are that this proposal will improve the health care available to the currently uninsured part of the population. It will greatly reduce if not eliminate the cost shifting now resulting from uncompensated service to the uninsured population. It is universal care with continued private sector pressure for innovation and cost control, a system that fits our American style better than a government single payer system.

The above proposal depends on the cooperation and support of CMS, the federal agency within the U.S. Department of Health and Human Services. That agency can do enough of what's needed within existing laws to make the proposal work. The current Medicaid law is such a confusing mess with a variety of poorly meshing add-ons that have accumulated over the years that CMS has extraordinary flexibility in how it administers the federal side of the Medicaid program. It is unlikely that the CMS management in place as this is written in the fall of 2004 would cooperate with such a program. Their strategy is to use approval of Medicaid waivers as a device to get the states to agree to capping the federal share of big parts of the Medicaid program.

This shifts the risk of medical inflation from one shared between the federal government and the states to one that falls strictly on the states. This strategy is incompatible with using the Medicaid Program as a shared financial responsibility vehicle to solve the uninsured problem. If this continues to be the CMS attitude, then we need a program that avoids using Medicaid waivers.

Such a program would be a three-way sharing of the financial responsibility with the states, the employers and the individuals being the three partners. Lacking the federal partner, the program could not be as generous. And I have reservations about whether it would work well enough to be worth doing. There are ways that the cost of a government health insurance program can be held down, absent federal involvement and federal regulations that increase costs. An obvious way to start is to limit drug availability to the cheapest one or two drugs in each class — a closed formulary.

People who wanted a different, more expensive drug could pay the difference between their choice and the one on the formulary. Higher deductible and co-payments could be used. The HSA concept could be used with the addition of the feature described above of having the individual HSA account go into debt with the debt to be repaid by a percentage withheld from the individual's paycheck, possibly with the state sharing some of the risk if the amounts got impossibly large.

Even if Medicaid can't be used, it might be possible to get some federal participation by using the Child Health Program (CHIP) where most states already have an enhanced eligibility component in place and approved by the feds. To do this there might have to be a state funds only transition program to deal with the anti-crowd-out provision in the federal law.

Considerable creativity will be necessary to structure this kind of a universal care program whether it is a four-way partnership involving the Medicaid program or a three-way partnership not involving the federal government. If the federal government will cooperate, the four-way partnership is the better way to go. For either proposal to be successful in anything more that the very short term, it must be coupled with a serious effort to control costs. If it is not, medical inflation rising at two or three times other costs will cause the program to be a source of financial instability for all the partners. For this reason, I will oppose either version of this program in the Wyoming Legislature in the absence of effective reforms, including some of those outlined in this book, to control costs.

Successful reform of our health care system is both necessary and possible. This book has discussed many of the reforms needed. These reforms will happen only if the public demands them, does its part, and puts pressure on the providers, the employers, and the legislatures of the several states to act. If we do not act, we will drift into an acute crisis as the private financing of our health care system fails. The response to an acute crisis is likely to be an ill-conceived national system that will do disastrous damage to the quality of our health care.

The time for action is now.

Chapter 13, Footnotes

(1) P.L. 108-173

(2) Richard Cauchi, NCSL Health Program, "2004 State Legislation on Health Savings Accounts and Medical Savings Accounts," July 12, 2004, page 1.

(3) George C. Halvorson and George J. Isham, Epidemic of Care, Jossey-Bass, 2003, pages 41 and 42.

(4) Halvorson and Isham, Ibid, pages 184 and 185.

(5) John E. McDonough, "Health Care for All," presentation at NCSL annual meeting, July 21, 2004.

(6) Kathryn A. Phillips et al., "Use of Preventive Services by Managed Care Enrollees: an Updated Perspective," Health Affairs, January/February 2000, Vol. 19, No. 1, page 106.

(7) The Economist, "A survey of health-care finance," "Wasting disease, A tale of poor quality an inefficiency," July 17, 2004, pages 13 & 14.

(8) $1,992 vs. $4,887 per capita in purchasing power parity international dollars (PPP$). OECD data converted to PPP$. Uwe E. Reinhardt, Peter S. Hussey and Gerard F. Anderson, "U.S. Health Care Spending in An International Context," Health Affairs, May/June 2004, page 11.

(9) The Economist, Ibid, pages 13-14.

(10) David M. Cutler, Your Money or Your Life, Oxford University Press, 2004, page 105.

(11) Cutler, Ibid, pages 100-113.

(12) Cutler, Ibid, page 112.

(13) The Economist, Ibid, page 16.

(14) Vanessa Furhmans, The Wall Street Journal, "Health Insurer to Target Scans for Cost Cuts," August 19, 2004, pages B1 and B2.

(15) See "Why the Rich Live Longer," Forbes, June 7, 2004, page 113-114. Forbes was reporting on a series of papers by Linda Gottfredson, a sociologist at the University of Delaware, and psychologist Ian Deary of the University of Edinburgh.

(16) The Wall Street Journal, "Health and Poverty," August 27, 2004, page A12.

(17) Census Bureau data cited in The Wall Street Journal, Ibid, page A12.

Appendix 1

COMPENDIUM OF TIPS TO SAVE MONEY AND IMPROVE HEALTH

Advertised Prescription Drugs: Be wary of the prescription drugs heavily advertised on TV. Their price will be increased by the cost of the TV advertising. Also, from what I've seen, often the most heavily advertised drugs are not as effective as others in their class. They have to be advertised because they aren't good enough to sell themselves. Don't go asking your doctor for one just because you saw it on TV. When you do ask about one, be careful to come across as asking your doctor's honest opinion, rather than demanding the drug. Sometimes in our litigious society the doctor will take the attitude that the customer is always right and give you what you want which may not be the best choice.

Antibiotic Drugs: Always take the full course of an antibiotic drug unless some serious side effect happens, in which case consult your doctor. With antibiotics the full course is needed to ensure the drug gets the job done and you don't have a relapse. Taking the full course also helps prevent the development of drug resistant bugs.

Antibiotic resistance: The development of antibiotic resistance is a major long term health concern. Microbes have shown an amazing ability to evolve resistance to our antibiotics. The early antibiotics that were wonder drugs when they first came out are now often ineffective. The use of antibiotics in cases where they are not effective (e.g. against viral diseases like most colds and influenza) is a practice that should be stopped not just because it wastes money (which it does), but primarily because it contributes to the development of resistance. I am also concerned about the use of low levels of antibiotics in animal feeds, a common practice with confined feeding operations (the practice is common with cattle and almost universal with chicken and hogs).

Alternative Medicine: It can work, see faith healing discussed below, but beware of treatments that may have bad side effects or interfere with needed medical care. Some treatments that can be classified as alternative medicine, like massage therapy, can provide useful symptomatic relief. Others, like chiropractic, are gradually picking up effective treatments from scientific medicine and becoming more useful in consequence. Much of alternative medicine, however, is harmless quackery and a danger only to your wallet.

Automatic External Defibrillator (AED): These are devices designed to restart a stopped heart by administering an electric shock to the chest. They work like the equipment in hospitals for just that job. They are much more effective than the standard closed chest CPR, although like CPR they have to be used promptly before the victim's brain starts to die from lack of oxygen. They are designed to be operated by an amateur. They are starting to appear in malls and stores and other places where people gather in numbers. They may even become available for home use. They should be operated by someone who has had some simple training, although in an emergency I think an untrained person could probably read the instructions and get the job done. If you want to do a public service, take the course in how to use them (consult your local Heart Association or Red Cross), and learn where the AEDs are located in places like your local mall. Some day you might save a life.

Back Problems: Welcome to the club; as many as four adults out of five eventually have back problems. After two or three million years of evolution we still aren't fully adapted to walking upright. Being overweight, being in poor shape due to a sedentary life style and poor posture can contribute to the problem, but people have problems without these risk factors. Appropriate use of ice and heat can help — consult any reputable family medicine book. Massage therapy can help relieve symptoms. Physical therapy can be very useful especially if the problem is a muscle sprain or spasm. I would go to a physical therapist first with a back problem, providing state law allowed it as most now do. The physical therapist will refer you to a doctor for medical evaluation if she thinks there might be something going on that needs medical evaluation. Often the physical therapist can give you a set of exercises that, if done faithfully, can go a long way to reduce the frequency and severity of problems. Be very wary of back surgery. It should be a last resort. Sometimes it is necessary to solve the problem, but too often it doesn't improve things or makes them worse. I would always get a second opinion before back surgery.

Blood Pressure: High blood pressure is a major silent killer that shows no overt symptoms. It is a major risk factor for a number of important killers including heart attacks and strokes. Get your blood pressure checked every now and then and go to your doctor if it's consistently high. Follow his recommendations faithfully including taking any drugs he prescribes. One word of caution, blood pressure wanders all over the place depending on the testing conditions, especially what you were doing immediately before the test. You need to be calm and relaxed when your blood pressure is taken. If just before you took a blood pressure test on the supermarket machine, you spent a minute chasing a two year old who was making a break for freedom, don't be surprised by a high reading. All it means is you're normal.

Blood Pressure Home Monitor: Probably a good idea if you have a blood pressure problem. It costs about fifty bucks at a good discount store. It can give you a warning of a problem before your doctor will have the opportunity to pick it up at a check up. If diet and lifestyle changes are an important part of your strategy for controlling blood pressure, it can give you important feedback on how well your are doing. They are quite reliable and easy to use, but you do have to pay attention to the testing conditions.

CT (Computed Tomography) Scans: A very useful diagnostic test that unfortunately carries some long term risk for the patient. The images that the CT scan can provide of what is really going on inside a patient's brain, chest, or abdomen are truly amazing and can be a big help in making a diagnosis or planning a treatment. Unfortunately the CT scan uses a lot of ionizing radiation. My home medical guide (The Harvard Medical School Family Health Guide, Simon & Schuster, 1999) shows the radiation from a single CT scan of the head and body as 1,100 times that of an arm or leg X-ray and 110 times that of a dental X-ray. As reported earlier (see Chapter 2) experts have pegged the risk of a single CT scan causing a fatal cancer as between 1 in 2,000 and 1 in 2,500. I caution these numbers vary with individual circumstances, may improve over time as the technology improves. I would recommend avoiding CT scans unless there is a real medical need for them. They are an unreasonable risk to take just to protect your doctor from legal liability. When used as a screening in a healthy patient, the risk from the scan may well exceed the benefit in finding unsuspected problems. You have to protect your own interests here — I have found too many doctors simply ignore the long term risks from ionizing radiation.

Diets: Be skeptical of the most recent fad, especially if what's being promoted involves spending money on special products or over-the-counter drug remedies. There is no magic bullet. Any reasonable diet will work if it effectively restricts your calories, but you have to stick with it and not cheat. Extra exercise also helps. And once you've finished the diet, you can't go back to the old habits that got you in trouble in the first place. There is some evidence that the popular Adkins diet works better than most, but the fundamental keys remain the same — restrict calories, get exercise, and stick with it.

End of Life Care: We can do a lot to improve the quality of life people have during their last few months of life. A lot depends on how well the individuals and their immediate families understand what's going on and what the realistic options are. Hospice is a good choice for those with some diseases (like many cancers) where the course of the disease is relatively predictable, but many diseases are not adequately predictable. Doctors sometimes have a very human reluctance to discuss the options frankly. This is understandable, but it can keep the patients and their families from making the best of a bad situation. A good book to consult on this issue is <u>Sick to Death and Not Going to Take It Anymore! Reforming Health Care for the Last Years of Life</u>, by Joanne Lynn (University of California Press, 2004) one of the California/Milbank books on health and the public.

Exercise: Do it, it's good for you. It will improve your health and make you feel better. Within reason, the evidence is the more the better, but the evidence also shows that even moderate exercise is quite beneficial. Our ancestors got lots of exercise of necessity; we evolved adapted to exercise. Our current sedentary life style is unnatural and consequently unhealthy. The key to an exercise program you will stick with is to pick exercise that you enjoy. Some people like to walk, some jog, some like to swim or do water exercises, some play sports, some, believe it or not, even like to run on treadmills. The important thing is to do it regularly.

Faith Healing: If you really believe, it can help or even cure some illnesses. It can be particularly helpful with psychosomatic illnesses. It can help with chronic conditions where the sufferer has to live with a level of discomfort or even pain. In this modern era pseudo science is as often the source of the faith as religion. The placebo effect is real. The trouble comes if a person ignores a medical condition that needs real medical care to be cured.

Heart Attacks: Heart disease is the major killer of both men and women. Screening for risk factors and action when one shows up is important. Learn the symptoms for a heart attack. When you have one, getting prompt medical attention can save your life. The symptoms in women can be different than those in men and can be harder to recognize.

HIV/AIDS: A fatal venereal disease. HIV is the virus. When it develops enough symptoms the person is said to have AIDS. A person with the HIV virus will develop and die from AIDS unless something else kills them first. Unprotected sex is the most common means of transmission, but other means are possible including especially sharing of needles (often done in abuse of injected illegal drugs), and mother to baby transmission. Health care workers are at risk if they come in contact with patients' blood or body fluids. They have learned to take careful precautions (HIV is not the only virus that can be transmitted this way). The risks of catching HIV vary with different populations and naturally go up the more sexual partners a person has and the more promiscuous the relevant culture is. So called "safe sex" (using condoms) provides a high degree of protection, but the only absolutely certain ways of preventing HIV infection are abstinence and mutual monogamy.

Herbs and Herbal Remedies: Usually harmless and sometimes beneficial or tasty, but some common sense precautions are in order. Like many things, they can be dangerous if taken in excessive quantities or, with some, for too long a period. Some can decrease fertility. Some will interact with various prescription and over-the-counter drugs either reducing or enhancing the effect of the drug or causing toxic effects. Herbal teas, if drunk in large quantities can, not surprisingly, have the same effect as the herbs themselves. A reasonable precaution if you want to take an herbal supplement or quantities of an herb itself is to look it up and see what the possible side effects, risks, and interactions are and be governed accordingly.

Another factor to consider is that the regulatory scheme for herbal supplements is different from that for drugs. There is less regulatory restraint on the kinds of health claims that can made about them. This is not intended as a criticism of our regulatory system. Many of us take at least some herbs because we like the taste in certain foods (for example garlic or herbal teas) so the regulatory system should be different.

Hype: Be wary of media hype of medical problems. The media has chronic trouble separating the esoteric, one in a million chances from the every day real risks that you should worry about. The problem is this distorts people's perceptions of what the real risks are. Too often they spend too much time and effort on preventing the unlikely risks and die from their untreated high blood pressure.

An additional problem is that sometimes new medical treatments and drugs are hyped without adequate qualification as to what their proper uses, contraindications, and risks are. In medicine as in many areas of life there is often a second side to the story and if it sounds to good to be true, it usually isn't true. The problem is that in medicine there can be real breakthroughs and it takes a careful professional who stays up to date to separate the real miracles from the false ones.

Generic Drugs: Unless you have a specific reason not to, always buy the generic for a prescription drug, if there is one. Due to government regulations the active ingredients should be the same and only rarely will the form, preparation, or inert ingredients make a difference. Just asking for the generic is not always adequate. In at least one common situation (high blood pressure) the generic often the most useful (a diuretic) is not a generic to many of the brand name drugs prescribed. Do pay a little attention to the prices; especially when the generics first come out and there isn't yet enough competition they can approach or even exceed the brand names in price. Also, if you are getting drugs from Canada, check prices. Their generics can be more expensive than American ones.

Injuries & Sprains: When you need wrap for an athletic injury or a sprain, go to your local feed store and buy Vet wrap. It's a lot cheaper than the wrap for people sold in the drug stores and for all practical purposes it's the same product.

Mad Cow Disease: A prion disease of cattle related to Creutzfeldt-Jacob disease in humans, scrapie in sheep, and chronic wasting disease in deer and elk. The disease is spread by cannibalism. The British were turning their cows into cannibals by feeding them meat and bone meal derived from diseased dead cows. They had a massive outbreak and proved it is possible, but very difficult, to transmit the disease to humans. The human disease, Creutzfeldt-Jacob disease, has a very low incidence of spontaneous occurrence possibly arising from accidental misfolding of prion proteins at the molecular level. It is possible the same occurs in cows although the rate should be very low as the incidence increases with age and cows rarely live beyond ten or twelve years. Using the British experience as of 2003, I calculated that if we had as many as ten bovine cases a year in the United States and took no precautions, we should expect to transmit a case from cows to humans once every 142 years. At this rate we may have had one or two human cases in the United States since we became a country. We now take precautions, including excluding brain and spinal cord material where the prions mostly are from the food supply, so this significantly overstates the risk. Put the risk of catching mad cow disease in your mental file of things you don't have to worry about.

Moderation: "Moderation in all things." This was my grandmother's favorite saying and remains the best advice I've seen on diet and lifestyle issues.

Parking Lots: In a big parking lot, take the first spot you see rather than circling looking for a "better" (closer in) spot. I know its un-American, but on average you'll save time and a little gas and the extra walking is good for you.

Prescription Drugs: Understand why your doctor has prescribed a drug for you and be sure you understand his instructions. Some drugs have to be taken with food, others on an empty stomach. Ask your doctor what you should do if you forget a dose. Some drugs can be taken on an as needed basis. Others, like antibiotics, have to be taken until the prescribed amount is finished. Still others, like ones for chronic conditions like blood pressure need to be taken essentially permanently.

Prescription Drugs 2: Try to be as faithful as possible in taking drugs your doctor has prescribed for chronic conditions like high blood pressure, diabetes, or high cholesterol. They really do prevent or delay life threatening conditions. In the long run they will give you a longer, healthier life and save you money.

Hospice: A good choice for many people with terminal illnesses, especially ones like cancer. A well run hospice can help you avoid aggressive care that can ruin the quality of what life you have left and amount to high tech torture as well as be very expensive. Probably not an appropriate choice if the illness is one where aggressive care can get you by this episode and give you significantly more time of quality life.

Radiation: The conventional wisdom is that all ionizing radiation carries some risk. Ionizing radiation is radiation strong enough to create ions; nuclear radiation and X-rays are examples. We cannot escape some radiation; all of us are exposed to radiation from the decay of natural radioactive elements and from cosmic sources. Conventional belief is the amount of risk from radiation is proportional to the dosage. There is some controversy about whether very low doses of radiation really have any risk. The risks possible are so low that I doubt this will be settled anytime soon. Simple X-rays (arm and leg, chest, dental) have so little radiation that I would not be concerned unless you get excessive numbers. Some of the more complicated X-ray studies and some scans, especially the CT scans, use enough radiation I would be concerned and would avoid them unless there is a real medical reason. This is one area where defensive medicine due to our tort liability system is harming patients. Once caution, there are scientific and engineer advances in this area. Over time we are learning to do the same task with less radiation so a risk that is a concern now may be much less of a concern in a few years.

Second Opinions: Not for everyday use due to the cost, second opinions can be very useful in certain circumstances. Life threatening illness and situations where the prospective treatments include measures that are risky, likely to produce disability, or very expensive all are circumstances where a second opinion may be appropriate. Your doctor may be very good, but he's human and someone else may pick up something he has missed or have a different perspective on the treatment options. Remember the discussion in Chapter 4 that the state of medical knowledge is so complex that no person can keep up on all the advances. Each circumstance is unique, so you have to use judgment and common sense in deciding if a second opinion is needed.

Small Pox: Historically one of mankind's worst enemies. The eradication of natural small pox is one of public health's crowning achievements. The only real risk now is that some government kept an illicit stock and some terrorist organization will get its hands on it. Apparently during the cold war the Soviet Union created a large stockpile of weaponized small pox. We must hope it has all been destroyed. In the absence of a proven threat, be very wary of small pox vaccination campaigns. The current vaccine has a significant risk of serious side effects particularly when given to an adult who has not previously been vaccinated (most people born since 1979). The vaccination does wear off after a while (12 years is a common estimate, but the process is probably gradual). If we ever do have a modern outbreak, follow instructions from authorities very carefully. Small pox is very contagious and has a high mortality rate and a high rate of complications. It may have killed as much as 90% of some native American populations that had not been previously been exposed to the disease. A real small pox outbreak would be one situation where the media hype would probably understate the seriousness of the problem.

Soft Drinks: There are a surprising number of calories in the typical can of pop. I found switching from regular soft drinks to the diet ones was one of the easiest ways to cut down on calories and sugars. You do have to get used to a little different taste.

Strokes: A major killer that can also disable. Learn the symptoms of a stroke. If you, or more likely someone you love, shows symptoms of a stroke, act immediately. Call 911 for an ambulance unless you have a better plan thought out. The victim needs to be under expert care in a hospital at once. There is clot busting medication that if given in the first hour after the stroke can destroy the offending clot and prevent all or most of the damage from the stroke. Unfortunately the victim has to be tested first because 12% of the strokes are caused by bleeding rather than clots and the medication would make those strokes worse, possibly killing the patient.

Swimming and Water Exercise: A good form of exercise for anyone who enjoys it. It could be especially useful for someone who is overweight or has arthritis. The water partly supports you and relieves a lot of the weight bearing stress on joints.

Tobacco: Don't use it. It is a risk factor for almost every possible health problem and the major cause of lung cancer. If you do use it, quitting is probably the most important single thing you can do to improve your health. And support those of us legislators who want to not just tax it, but tax the hell out of it. Running the price up with taxes (or any other way) does encourage people to quit and helps keep young people from starting. Only a teenager is dumb enough to start smoking or chewing.

Tuberculosis: Historically a major killer that public health and modern medicine have largely beaten back. The disease is still present, mostly in homeless and drug abusing populations although sometimes someone in the general population catches it. If we are incautious and if the micro-organism involved develops resistance to the drugs used as it seems to be gradually doing, this disease could come back a be a major killer again. If you ever get it, treat it as a major medical emergency and follow doctors orders carefully.

Vaccines: Possibly the best preventive medicine available. Make sure the children in your family get all the recommended vaccinations. We are getting too lax about childhood vaccinations. As a result there is a risk the diseases may come back as whooping cough (pertussis, the P in the DPT vaccine) currently is. There are a number of vaccinations adults need under certain conditions including ones for tetanus, pneumonia, flu, and hepatitis A and B. Pay attention to the recommendations and whether they include you. Periodically check them as recommendations do change as new vaccines are developed or new medical problems arise. The 2004 flu vaccine shortage hopefully will be a one time problem, but we need to rethink our vaccine manufacturing strategy.

Vitamins and Vitamin Supplements: These can be useful in certain circumstances. A healthy person with a balanced diet should get an adequate supply of most vitamins without needing an artificial supplement. However in certain situations taking vitamin supplements is medically indicated. Follow you doctor's orders. Also, know what the recommendations are if you might become pregnant. Like most things it is possible to get in medical trouble by overdoing some vitamins; use a little common sense. It is also possible to waste money taking too many vitamins.

Weight Loss Pills: Especially when heavily advertised, Quack, Quack, Quack. With many of these, the only weight loss is likely to be in your wallet. However, there is always the possibility of a scientific advance in this area. If it happens, some drug company is going to make a lot of money.

Appendix 2

SUMMARY OF HEALTH CARE COST ANALYSES

I have encountered a number of different summaries of how health care costs divide into various categories and how the categories are contributing to the rise in health care costs. Since understanding where the cost increases are coming from and how much they are is a first step in controlling costs, these are of considerable interest. I think the underlying numbers are the same or similar for most of the analyses, but there are significant differences in what categories are used to define the costs. Some summaries are more useful than others in figuring out what to do about the problem. I include in this appendix, summaries from a number of sources so the reader can draw his own conclusions.

I. The Henry J. Kaiser Family Foundation,
    Chartbook, May 2002[1]

Distribution of National Health Expenditures by Type of Service

The figures in the first two columns are the percentage of the total expenditures in each category in that year. The third column is the percentage that item is of the increase in costs over the decade.

Type	1900	2000	Percentage of 1990/2000 Increase
Hospital Care	36.5%	31.7%	26.2%
Physician/clinical services	22.6	22.0	21.4
Prescription drugs	5.8	9.4	13.5
Nursing home care	7.6	7.1	6.5
Home health care	1.8	2.5	3.3
Other personal health care	13.3	14.3	15.4
Other health spending	12.4	13.0	13.7

II. PricewaterhouseCoopers (PWC) "The Factors Fueling Rising Healthcare Costs," April, 2002[2]

PricewaterhouseCoopers estimated the overall average increase in health insurance premiums for large employers from 2001 to 2002 at 13.7 percent. They point out that this is higher than the rise in medical costs measured by the federal government. It includes any rise in insurance administrative costs, but it primarily reflects benefit costs. I point out that these are inflated above pure medical inflation by cost shifting from government programs and the uninsured (see Chapter 6). The percentages in the table are the PWC estimates of the percentage each factor contributes to the total growth. They are not the percentage each is of total expenses.

Category	Percent of Total Increase
General inflation (CPI)	18%
Drugs, medical devices & med advances	22%
Rising provider expenses*	18%
Increased consumer demand**	15%
Government mandates & regulation	15%
Litigation & risk management***	7%
Other	5%

   * Hospitals negotiating higher payments

 ** Aging population, increased preventive and diagnostic expenses, shift away from less expensive managed care products, demand for expensive treatments.

*** Lawsuits, malpractice premiums, increased defensive medicine.

III. Center for Studying Health System Change, reporting Milliman USA Health Cost Index[3]

The table reports the percentage share each factor contributes to overall health care spending growth based on claims increases faced by private insurers.

Category	1999	2000	2001
Physician services	30%	34%	28%
Prescription drugs	34%	27%	21%
Hospital inpatient	5%	7%	14%
Hospital outpatient	31%	32%	37%

IV. BlueCross BlueShield Association, "Inpatient Expenditure Growth Contributions"[4]

This table shows the contribution each of the factors made to the growth in expenditures for a large national health insurance plan over the period 1998 to 2000. The 2000 data were compared to 1998 data to arrive at the percentage increases.

Medical wages	20%
Hospital technology	19%
Hospital market structure	18%
Hospital underutilization	15%
Income	10%
Physician market	5%
Hospital fragmentation	4%
Population	3%
Population morbidity	3%
Nurse shortage	2%
State regulations	1%

BlueCross BlueShield Association, "Contributions to private insurance spending growth, 2000"[5]

Hospital inpatient	31%
Prescription drugs	29%
Physician	28%
Hospital outpatient	12%

BlueCross BlueShield Association, "Relative Importance of Outpatient Cost Driver Categories"[6]

This chart was developed by the Lewin Group for BlueCross BlueShield. It shows the results of a regression analysis on data from a large national private (commercial) health insurer. The percentages show the increase over the period 1998 to 2000.

Provider market structure	35%
Treatment patterns and technology	18%
General price inflation	18%
Physician & specialist supply	11%
Demographics and general economic conditions	7%
Provider payment	4%
Health care regulation	4%
Provider operating costs	3%

V. Council of State Governments, reporting data from Health Care Financing Administration (HCFA), U.S. Department of Health and Human Services data[7]

The table shows how HCFA reports the nation's health care dollar was spent in 1998 and is in percentages. This is total spending, not increase in spending.

Category	1998 Percent of Total Spending
Hospital care	33.3%
Physician services	20.0%
Prescription drugs	7.9%
Nursing home care	7.6%
Program administration and net cost	5.0%
Other spending	26.2%

VI. "Rising Medicaid Costs," the Kaiser Commission on Medicaid and the Uninsured[8]

The table shows the factor states reported as among the "top three" increasing Medicaid spending. The figures are the number of states reporting the factor in the top three. The numbers add to 82 percent of the total possible, so there were a scattering of other factors reported.

Factor	Number of States Reporting
Pharmacy	44
Enrollment	39
Cost of health services	28
Long-term care	15

VII. Sources of Payment for Health Care, CMS, Office of the Actuary[9]

Note this summary shows private sources as responsible for 54 percent of the health care spending in the U.S. with governmental sources at 46 percent. I am aware of other summaries that put the governmental share over 50 percent, but these count tax deductions as a governmental expenditure. It is not clear in this analysis whether local government employee health care expenditures are counted as governmental or private. The figures are for 2002.

Note that the figures are for expenditures. In most states both the Medicare and Medicaid programs pay significantly less than the cost of service with the resulting deficit cost shifted to the private sector as a hidden tax (see Chapter 6, Cost Shifting). This suggests that the governmental share of the total volume of medical care is significantly larger than its share of expenditures, but I have never seen this quantified.

Private

Private health insurance	35%
Out-of-pocket	14%
Other private	5%
Total private	54%

Federal

Medicare	17%
Medicaid, federal share	10%
Other federal	6%
Total federal	33%

State

Medicaid, state share	7%
Other state	6%
Total State	13%

Appendix 2, Footnotes

(1) The Henry J. Kaiser Family Foundation, Trends and Indications in the Changing Health Care Marketplace, Chartbook, May 2002, pages 10 & 11. Kaiser authors' calculations based on data from the Centers for Medicare and Medicaid Services (CMS), Office of the Actuary, National Health Statistics Group, posted on CMS website.

(2) PricewaterhouseCoopers, "The Factors Fueling Rising Healthcare Costs," April 2002, prepared for the American Association of Health Plans, pages 2 and 3.

(3) Center for Studying Health System Change, Data Bulletin, "Tracking Health Care Costs," No. 22, September 2002. The source for the data is "Milliman U.S.A. Health Cost Index ($0 deductible)."

(4) Joel Hay, Sharon Forest and Mireille Goetghebeur, "Executive Summary Hospital Costs in the U.S.," prepared for the BlueCross BlueShield Association, October 15, 2002, page 8. Included in "What's Behind the Rise: A Comprehensive Analysis of Healthcare Costs," published by the BlueCross BlueShield Association.

(5) Sharon Forest, Mireille Goetghebeur and Joel Hay, "Forces Influencing Hospital Costs in the United States," prepared for the BlueCross BlueShield Association, October 16, 2002, page 30. Included in "What's Behind the Rise: A Comprehensive Analysis of Healthcare Costs," published by the BlueCross BlueShield Association. Figures are adapted from the BlueCross BlueShield Report, 2002

(6) The Lewin Group, Inc, "Study of Healthcare Outpatient Cost Drivers," prepared for BlueCross BlueShield Association, pages 27 and 28. Included in "What's Behind the Rise: A Comprehensive Analysis of Healthcare Costs," published by the BlueCross Blue Shield Association.

(7) Council of State Governments, Health Policy Forum, "Summation Report, Prescription Drugs: Cost, Pricing and Innovation," undated flyer. Source reported, Health Care Financing Administration, U.S. Department of Health and Human Services.

(8) Adapted from a presentation by Stuart H. Altman to the National Conference of State Legislatures Spring Meeting, Boston, Mass., April 2003. Source is the Kaiser Commission on Medicaid and the Uninsured Survey of Medicaid officials in the 50 states and D.C., conducted by Health Management Associates, June 2002.

(9) Office of the Actuary, Center for Medicare and Medicaid Services (CMS), U.S. Department of Health and Human Services, as reported in Governing, The Magazine of States and Localities, August 2004, page 53.

INDEX

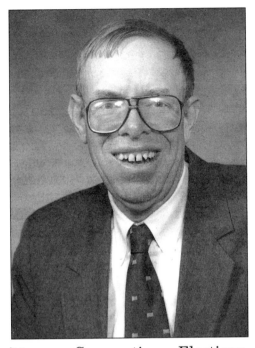

Senator Charles Scott was first elected to the Wyoming Legislature in 1978 and has served ever since. He served four years in the House and moved to the Senate after the 1982 election. Since 1993 he has been chairman of the committee that is responsible for health legislation, The Committee on Labor, Health and Social Services. Before that he was chairman of a temporary Select Health Committee and the committee which is responsible for insurance legislation, the Committee on Corporations, Elections, and Political Subdivisions. He has sponsored 43 bills that have become law.

From 2001 to 2004, Charles Scott served one year as Chair and two years as Vice Chair of the Health Committee of the National Conference of State Legislatures and currently serves on their Medicaid Task Force. He is a member of the steering committee of the Reforming States Group, a voluntary national association supported by the Milbank Foundation of state legislators and executives interested in health care issues. He is a member of the Advisory Board of the United States Cochrane Center.

Charles Scott earns his living as President of the Bates Creek Cattle Company, a small business which provides health insurance for its employees. He and his wife Elaine, a retired physical therapist, live on the ranch near Casper, Wyoming with their son, daughter-in-law and new granddaughter.

Scott is a graduate of Harvard College and has an MBA from the Harvard Business School. Before returning to the family ranch, he worked five years for the federal government in Washington, D.C., first for the Department of Health, Education and Welfare and then the Environmental Protection Agency.